Putting Chronic Fatigue To Rest
Treating Chronic Fatigue and Chronic Fatigue Syndrome with Maharishi Ayurveda

About the Author

Dr Kumuda Reddy has been practicing medicine for nearly forty years. She has developed a very informative website called "allhealthyfamily.com" which is dedicated to bringing the knowledge of the unlimited scope of Maharishi Ayurvedic Medicine. It is comprehensive, holistic and compatible with Conventional medicine.

Dr Reddy completed her residency and fellowship at Mt.Sinai Hospital, New York. She was the Medical Director of Maharishi Vedic Center in Bethesda, Maryland and a former faculty member of Albany Medical College. She was the Medical Director of Maharishi Rejuvenation Center in Thailand and travels extensively offering consultations across the globe.

Currently she is dividing her time between India and the US and is helping with expansion of Maharishi Ayurveda Globally.

Dr. Reddy, through her practice, books and lectures conveys this simple message, "that we are one with nature." Because of our intimate connection to nature and the entire cosmos, we need natural and holistic medicine. It is the need of our time. No other medicine has proven to be as natural, comprehensive, time-tested and holistic as Maharishi Ayurveda.

Dr. Reddy believes that the best way to avoid suffering and ill-health is to "avert the danger which has not yet come." This is the basic principle of prevention from the ancient Vedic tradition of health care. The earlier we start the better.

Taking this to heart, Dr. Reddy has co-authored several books.

Forever Healthy – Introduction to Maharishi Ayurveda Health Care
For a Blissful Baby – Healthy and Happy Pregnancy with Maharishi Vedic Medicine
Conquering Chronic Disease – Through Maharishi Vedic Medicine
Golden Transition – Menopause Made Easy through Maharishi Vedic Medicine
Living life free from pain – Treating Arthritis, Joint Pain Muscle Pain and Fibromyalgia with Maharishi Ayurveda
Super Healthy Kids - A Parents Guide to Maharishi Ayurveda
Ayurvedic Cooking Made Easy - 100+ Recipes for a Healthy You

Dr. Reddy has also co-authored a book of stories from the Upanishads entitled "All Love Flows to the Self" and a series of children's stories called the Timeless Wisdom series based on traditional Indian stories that she first heard from her grandmother. Dr. Reddy believes these stories will help educate children in the positive, nourishing and practical values that are so important for their health and happiness.

She has appeared on several radio and TV shows. Dr. Reddy has been contributing health articles to the local news magazines and papers. In addition to her life as a medical doctor, writer and speaker, Dr. Reddy is a wife, mother and an active community leader with dedication to bring this holistic health and peace to every family in the world.

At your bookstore or from the publisher:

Samhita Productions
College Park, Maryland
www.allhealthyfamily.com

Putting Chronic Fatigue To Rest

Treating Chronic Fatigue and Chronic Fatigue Syndrome
with Maharishi Ayurveda

by

Kumuda Reddy, M.D.

With Paul Stokstad

Samhita Productions

College Park, Maryland

Published by
Samhita Productions
College Park, Maryland

Book Design and Composition - Pixint (www.pixint.com)
Printed in the United States of America.

ISBN- 9781439237960

Dedication

To Maharishi Mahesh Yogi, for giving us his vision of natural and holistic health in all areas of our lives.

Contents

xi

Foreword and Acknowledgment

It's my great joy to bring you this book on putting chronic fatigue to rest. I really don't know anybody who never had serious fatigue at one time or another. It is an automatic result of the stress and chaos of living in the modern world. And even though this book tells the story of chronic fatigue, the hero of the story is Maharishi Ayurveda also known as Maharishi vedic medicine (MVM) , or consciousness-based medicine. It brings to us the knowledge that we are a manifestation of nature--the Sanskrit term is prakriti -and we are also, in our inner nature, deeply connected to a field of pure consciousness, or purusha, from which all creation comes.

Since we are an aspect of manifest nature, we can embody beauty, splendor, dynamism, diversity, infinite intelligence and all the other qualities of nature. And since we are also an aspect of pure consciousness, we are also the unity, totality and infinite silence underlying the infinite dynamism of creation

Through consciousness-based medicine, we can begin to both experience and understand the totality of what we are, the full range of life from infinite silence to dynamic action. This experience enlivens, rejuvenates and enlightens.

Just as in the perspective of modern physics there is a gross level of observation of the natural world, a subtle perspective, an even subtler level and then the subtlest quantum or unified field level, your body has a gross, subtle, subtler and also a subtlest level of pure consciousness. Understanding this, from the health perspective, we are motivated to utilize health modalities that can influence our health on all levels, from the grossest to the subtlest.

The subtlest level, pure consciousness, is the basis, source and foundation of everything else, subtle to gross. The inner connection of the individual to the unmanifest, infinite pure consciousness level of their own existence can only be known by experience and not by intellectual understanding.

So, if you didn't understand all that I have just said, that's okay, it's not about understanding it at all, it's about experiencing it.

Maharishi Ayurveda, fortunately, is an experiential science. Every step of well being and healing that is experienced stays in your memory. And that becomes the basis for personal progression and transformation in the direction of good, better, best, and then perfect health.

The wellness that you then experience ranges throughout the different states of consciousness, intellect, emotions, mind, body, behavior and environment.

That is why this system of creating health can also be called enlightened health. With a fully enlightened intellect you can discriminate between what is healthy and non-healthy, what is in accord with the laws of nature or violating the laws of nature, what is good for you or what is not appropriate for you.

This is called removing "the mistake of the intellect" (Sanskrit - pragyaparadh) the idea that you are somehow disconnected from the totality of life. When you are enlightened, this mistake is removed, and your intellect will support your mind in a balanced way and it will make wise choices.

You may be wondering whether a medical system based on such a grand vision will be easy to follow. Will I be able to comply with it?

Will it give me quick results? The answer is that it is easy to do because the processes themselves are easy, enjoyable and natural. You will be quickly aware of success in the healing process, and you will soon take charge of your own recovery.

A physician is initially needed to help you start the program and reduce the complexity of the program to something that is both customized for you and easily accessible.

Results are often quite rapid. You will usually start feeling better almost immediately, and with the confidence that you then gain you will be able to take further steps.

This program brings hope to all through treatment of the immediate disorder, prevention of further imbalance, and lifetime maintenance of optimized health, which makes life both enjoyable and worth living.

This is enlightened health for enlightened living.

I would like to thank Paul Stokstad for helping put this book together. His sense of humor and playful analogies make this book both readable and accessible. I would also like to thank Vaidya Hemant Gupta, Linda Egenes, David Orme-Johnson, and many others who helped make this book possible.

And I thank you for taking the steps to make yourself as healthy as you can , so that you can fulfill your role in bringing as much happiness as possible into your life, thereby contributing to the health, happiness and enlightenment of your family, friends, community, and the whole world.

CHAPTER 1

Overview

Susan, age 53, a government official, came to me with complaints of extreme chronic fatigue. The fatigue had started about 10 years ago while she was going through a change in jobs and a divorce. It gradually got worse, and for the last year she had become extremely fatigued and felt that she was unable to cope with the job or her life.

She said, "I have lost the joy in my life, I feel I'm perpetually dragging my feet, even to do the smallest chore."

Along with the chronic fatigue she had developed, she had no energy to exercise. She had been experiencing a lot of stress and anxiety. She was also in the middle of a menopausal transition at the same time. She used to be an occasional smoker and had recently become a one pack a day smoker.

She started developing digestive problems early on, with gas, bloating, and gradual constipation. For the past three years, she had experienced constant heartburn, and symptoms of constipation alternating with diarrhea. In the last few months before seeing me she had had constant diarrhea, four to 5 bowel movements a day, and felt drained out, in more ways than one.

She was taking many over the counter preparations for heartburn and diarrhea, with little or no relief, and was also on Premarin (a hormone replacement). She also had started developing low back pain and joint

pain in the small bones of the hands and feet. She also had stiffness and joint pain in the elbows, shoulders, hips and knees.
I guess that we could say that Susan was sick and sick of being sick. At least we know that she had a whole basketful of symptoms.

Her first statement when she came to my office was:

"I want to be as healthy as I can be, Doctor Reddy. I'm really tired of this tiredness, I would like to get rid of this diarrhea and quit smoking. I have tried several times to quit smoking. I feel extremely anxious and panicky. Can you please help me?"

At this point she had already been to several doctors. She was given a diagnosis of chronic fatigue, bordering on Chronic Fatigue Syndrome (CFS - the industrial strength version of chronic fatigue which is also known as Myalgic Encephalopathy - more on this later), irritable bowel syndrome, and arthritis, and many others. Howeverand this is the strange partshe had been worked up and investigated to the maximum, but her lab tests were normal, except for early osteoporotic changes in the spine.

That means that she had all of these symptoms, yet she was not sick, according to traditional allopathy medicine. None of the normal tests indicated that this lady was sick.

People like this have trouble being taken seriously. Sometimes their insurance companies don't want to pay, or employers fire them, because, after all, "the doctor says you aren't sick."

Something is wrong here. Why is she sick when her doctors can't find out why? At this point, the traditional physician starts to drift over to a diagnosis of psychosomatic causes. But before we take the same route let's look at some other possibilities.

Let's consider for a moment that the diagnostic and treatment systems we typically use may have limitations whereby we don't recognize the causes of some diseases, and therefore we are at a loss to identify and treat them.

Just like a radar system that can't recognize the outlines of a Stealth bomber, we may be unable to see and detect some problems until it is too late. On the other hand, the cause may turn out not to be terribly important. It may be that we are as if surveying the damage after the bomb has fallen and trying to figure out what kind of plane it was that dropped the bomb.

It may be more important to start rebuilding.

Just Tired, or Sick and Tired?

Patients like Susan have a wide variety of words or phrases they use to describe how they are doing: beat, tired out, bushed, dead tired, dog tired, weak as a kitten, etc. As physicians, we have to get a bit more specific, so we administer tests. These are a different kind of test: the kind you want to fail. There are many reasons why you might be tired, regardless of what you call it, and it's the doctor's job to eliminate all of the usual suspects first, before we throw your case into the Chronic Fatigue basket.

This is called exclusionary testing. There are quite a number of these, including complete blood count (tests for anemia, blood disorders, malignancies, viral infections, etc.), blood sedimentation rate (usually elevated when you are seriously ill, but not with CFS), routine chemistries (these can find diabetes mellitus, hepatitis, kidney failure), thyroid screen (thyroid imbalances can cause weakness and fatigue), thyroid antibodies (for thyroiditis), HIV antibody, rheumatoid factor (arthritis), antinuclear antibody (lupus), lyme disease antibodies, chest x-ray (infections, malignancies, sarcoidosis), urinalysis (various diseases).

Those are the nice tests, i.e.- non-invasive. Then we have lumbar puncture (tests for multiple sclerosis), upper and lower GI series (x-rays that can find duodenal or gastric ulcers, Crohn's disease, ulcerative colitis, et al.). There's more: bowel endoscopy, liver and spleen scan, bone marrow aspirate, lymph node biopsy, CT scan of the brain, and other things designed to find out if you have conditions like cancer, leukemia, tuberculosis, lymphoma, Hodgkin's disease, brain tumors, syphilis, and a bunch of ailments with long names, like reactive hyperplasia, toxoplasmosis, and cytomegalovirus.

As it turns out, there are over 200 medical conditions that have fatigue as a component. Did I mention the various kinds of sleep disorder, dietary deficiencies, Parkinson's disease, stress, and depression? Many of these ailments act almost exactly like Chronic Fatigue Syndrome. Multiple sclerosis has many CFS symptoms, yet it is not the same thing. Fibromyalgia also mirrors CFS in many ways, yet it's not a twin. Just a sick relative.

After you have failed all these tests and you still feel sick, you might start to wish to pass one of them, just so that you know what's wrong with you. Giving a name to your malady is somehow settling to the mind. At least you know what you are dealing with. And even that is a luxury that was denied Chronic Fatigue Syndrome sufferers for years.

If you failed all of those tests (that's good!) and you still have most of the following symptoms, you are a candidate for a diagnosis of Chronic Fatigue Syndrome:

- Mild fever
- Sore throat
- Painful lymph nodes
- Muscle weakness
- Muscle pain
- Prolonged fatigue after exercise
- Headaches
- Joint pain
- Neuropsychologic complaints
- Sleep disturbance
- Acute onset of symptoms

With CFS you have two out of three of the following:
- Low grade fever

- Throat inflammation
- Palpable or tender lymph nodes [1]

Of course, you may not have all of these symptoms, or even most of these symptoms. Maybe you don't have CFS, but you don't ever feel rested, you get up feeling unrefreshed, you drag through the day, you dream of at least one good night's sleep, and you find it hard to care about work, relationships, eating or doing anything.

So, you're not bad off, right?

Of course not, you're in an awful state, living a life of reduced capacity to enjoy, create and accomplish things. You deserve better. But you are simply deeply fatigued, not "sick" in a traditional sense. You have plain old chronic fatigue. On the other hand, if you have all of those symptoms and the bevy of other ailments that I mentioned above, you may have CFS. Neither one is much fun.

We need to make a clear distinction between these two conditions. Chronic fatigue is a serious problem, debilitating and discouraging. If you feel that you are always tired, and can't even seem to get rested, even after a full night's sleep, life becomes duller, accomplishment is less. Such fatigue certainly clouds your experience of life, and can even make you more accident prone, and probably more disease-prone, since poor psychological states apparently reduce immunity and invite illness. Your reaction time may suffer, reducing your driving skills, even to the level of an inebriated driver. But despite all that, you are just chronically fatigued, not yet suffering from CFS.

---

1. Copyright 1992, National Chronic Fatigue Syndrome Association, page 4

In this book I will discuss many modalities of treatment which can rapidly address the condition of chronic fatigue, and have a positive effect on CFS patients. But it would be misleading to indicate that these are the same conditions with the same degree of responsiveness to short-term treatment.

It's not that I don't believe that CFS sufferers can be treated successfully and even relieved of the symptoms of what most physicians consider an irreversible condition. It's just that CFS patients need to be even more patient than the chronically fatigued patient. They need more intensive help, monitored treatment, possibly under the auspices of one of the Chronic Disease Centers that I will be describing later.

In any case, let's look at how these fatigue conditions happen to nice people like you, or to people who at least used to be nice before they got so tired.

Chronic fatigue can arrive in a number of ways. You can have a poor diet, irregular work or sleeping schedules, stressful work and emotional environments. You may have various kinds of sleeping disorders, you may be recovering (or trying to recover) from a divorce, death of a spouse, child, parent, friend, or dealing with a change in employment, career setback, or even a career advancement that requires significant changes in your life. Or you may have some form of depression. There are lots of ways to get chronically tired. And it can be even more serious, if you have CFS.

If you have CFS, the obvious question is: how did I get it? Somehow we think if we can isolate the cause we may be able to identify a cure.

Unfortunately, there may be many roads that lead to the same result.

Even so, let's take a look at some of the current theories of how Chronic Fatigue Syndrome gets started, since, as it turns out, it is not only difficult to diagnose, it's origin is more difficult to pinpoint than the pot of gold at the end of the rainbow, and not as much fun if you find it.

First of all, maybe you are just depressed. Maybe it's all in your head. That's what your friends, your doctor and your boss are going to start thinking as soon as you come home with that stack of failed test papers. More doctors are alerted to CFS nowadays, but there is still a good chance that they will start looking at you funny and removing sharp objects from the room. And it's all because they can't find out what's wrong with you. You don't show up on their radar scope, so you must be weird. It couldn't be that the radar is ineffective or incomplete, now could it?

You didn't need a doctor to tell you that you were depressed. But it's not all a matter of making an attitude adjustment, since it could be that mild fever, sore throat, painful lymph nodes, muscle weakness, muscle pain, prolonged fatigue, headaches, joint pain, sleep disturbances has somehow got you down, not your attitude.

So what came first, the tired chicken or the sleepy egg? Clinically depressed people may feel like listless slugs, but they don't usually have night sweats, lymph node pain, sore throat and joint pain, like CFS patients. Plus, depressed people usually don't have fatigue like that of a CFS patient, which is "bone-crushing and flu-like."

When people with CFS spend time with friends, or do things that they usually enjoy, they still get a lot of enjoyment unlike depressed people. Folks with CFS want to try things, but get exhausted with minimal physical and mental activities. Fatigue does not improve with rest or sleep.

Confronted with this question, a number of theories have been proposed to explain how CFS happens. And it's not easy to find a solution to this question, because a cause would have to be pretty sophisticated to do everything that CFS does. If we were writing a job description for the cause of CFS, it would have to go something like this:

1. Must cause severe fatigue and exhaustion, plus : mild fever, sore throat, painful lymph nodes, muscle weakness, muscle pain, prolonged fatigue after exercise, headaches, joint pain, neuropsychological complaints, sleep disturbance, abdominal pain, difficulty with concentration and memory.
2. Must affect children and adults but rarely children under 5
3. Must affect women more than men (two out of three)
4. Must be debilitating.
5. Must cause immune dysfunction (usually "up-regulated" immunity... The immune system activated like crazy with no apparent reason. Victims feel sick all of the time. Your body thinks it's fighting something, but of course there is nothing there to fight, according to all of your tests)
6. Must cause sudden or gradual onset of disease

7. Must cause a wide variety of severity of the disease

8. Must afflict a higher percentage of people with asthma and/or allergies

9. Must have increased incidence within families.[2]

So who are the candidates for this job? Epstein-Barr syndrome, Coxsackie B virus, Herpes virus, Polio virus, hypothyroidism, encephalitis, AIDS and others have been investigated as possible causes. But all have been rejected for various reasons. One fascinating candidate, however, is a potential form of retrovirus, which is a unique virus that merges into the human genetic material, from where it expands its penetration into the host tissues through the normal processes of human DNA duplication.

This retrovirus may trigger the up-regulated immune system, which mobilizes to attack the invader, but the invader looks just like the host, so the immune system keeps attacking the host laying waste to the countryside (your body). Still, no such active agent has been isolated, and research continues.

Meanwhile, while the debates about cause go on, and the researchers call for more and more funding, patients continue to suffer, and little seems to be available to help them, other than to treat their symptoms.

There are plenty of people with the symptoms, too, so, if you have it, you are not alone. It is estimated that as many as one million people in the U.S. have a CFS-like condition.

---

2. The Doctor's Guide to Chronic Fatigue Syndrome,
   Bell, David S., Da Capo Press, 1995, pp. 201-202 [8]

Allopathic medicine has very little to offer. Main modality is cognitive behavioral therapy. It simply means self help to recognize you own weaknesses. They give nutritional supplements and advice you to attend support groups. Not much to speak of. There is no test for CFS. It is diagnosed by ruling out other problems.

Onto this stage steps Maharishi Ayurveda, with a completely different approach to resolving this apparent dilemma, an approach which seems to be working, despite the fact that the exact culprit behind Chronic Fatigue Syndrome has not been found. [3]

It may turn out that there is no culprit, of course. It may turn out that we have finally found an illness with no "active causative agent," an illness where you are just sick, without a specific cause. It could be an illness that is a general result of imbalances that have built up in the body over a period of years, and the lack of specific, medically testable irregularities associated with the illness may only result in throwing into question our testing or our model of what constitutes illness.

Through Maharishi Ayurveda, we often discover that there may be a wide variety of reasons why you got fatigued, depending on your lifestyle, body type (more on that soon), etc. The search for a single cause may obscure the individualized nature of your particular path to illness, and therefore cloud the prospects for effective, personalized treatment.

---

3. U.S. Center for Disease Control, CFS Demographics,
   http://chronicfatigue.about.com/health/chronicfatigue/library/cdc/blcdc_demo.htm

Causal agents are important, but even without a universal diagnostic marker, Maharishi Ayurveda can typically move straight to rejuvenation and cure, once we have eliminated a few of the obvious candidates for fatigue.

Once we have done that, we know that you are not fatigued due to a typical illness, and are simply in need of the deeply rejuvenative therapies of MVM. It's not that your condition is no longer serious, it's just a different kind of serious.

To understand just how serious it is, we have to backtrack a little, and show you when you started getting sick (and tired). It started long before you went to the doctor.

To do this we will discuss Maharishi Ayurveda(MVM), how it views the body, what you may have done to contribute to your condition, the course of your illness, the origins of fatigue itself, how diagnosis takes place in MVM, and its holistic treatment modalities that can put your imbalances to rest.

CHAPTER 2

The Big Picture

Now let's talk about you. What's happening right now, right where you are? What are the elements of your experience? You are sitting, standing, or lying down. You are surrounded by objects of various kinds. You are probably clothed, surrounded by air of (hopefully) a comfortable temperature. There may or may not be other people around you. You may subjectively be in one mood or another. You, might, actually, be feeling a bit fatigued. You are reading this book. These are the probable scenarios. There are exceptions, of course, but these are likely.

All of this seems obvious, but there is more to your situation than we normally consider. The other element, that completes the picture, is the fact that you are conscious. Your own consciousness adds something to the equation. If you leave the situation you are in, let's say the room that you are sitting in, more has left the room than a body. An observer has left.

What does all this mean, or matter? It's about consciousness. The fact that you are conscious brings a whole other element into the picture. We don't normally think of our own conscious nature as a phenomenon, but it is a very palpable experience that we all have, or at least a condition from which we function.

We experience personal consciousness in varying forms. Just like water takes varying forms of liquid, gas, or solid (ice), consciousness can evidently be experienced in different levels or modes. Some days we are alert and sharp; consciousness is full and strong. Maybe later in the day we get tired, and our alertness gets shadowed and dull. Then we sleep; consciousness is apparently absent. But then we dream.

Modern research has indicated that each of the states of consciousness, waking, sleeping, and dreaming have distinct corresponding physiological correlates. A physiologist can stand in the next room and with only breathing and EEG monitors hooked up to your body, tell without looking at you whether you are waking, sleeping or dreaming.

Imagine a view of life where the fact that you are awake, conscious and alive is considered the primary element of existence, not matter. Where your own conscious awareness or consciousness is the primary measure of your liveliness, not your heart or breathing rate.

Since we all experience various degrees of "consciousness'" depending on how well rested we are, what time of day it is, etc., the body, in this model, could be considered a successful organism if it supports maximum alertness, consciousness, or wakefulness.

In this view, fatigue would be seen as a substandard style of functioning of the body, and an enlightened state of mental functioning, as in "higher states of consciousness" would be considered optimal, or even more truly normal.

Most of allopathy medicine looks at the physical body as being primary, and the fact that you are conscious is an afterthought, a given. Allopathy medicine will note (somewhere on your chart) if you are unconscious, but that's about it.

But what happens to our view of the body if we look at it from the other direction? Starting from there, we end up with an entirely different model of physiological function, not to mention human potential. We're not mentioning human potential just now because first we have to get you out of that fatigue thing. But it is important, so more on that later.

Consciousness is where Maharishi Vedic Medicine gets its start. Maharishi Vedic Medicine (MVM) is based on a world view that consciousness is the primary constituent of creation, not matter. Now that might seem to be a radical perspective, if it weren't for the fact that some quantum physicists have long shared the same view, that the most fundamental field of existence is a unified field which evidently must be seen as a field of pure consciousness in order to account for the physical and energy-field phenomena that such physicists have discovered.

When you think about it, a truly comprehensive theory of the universe - which is something that all science would eventually dream of producing - would have to account for the fact that we are conscious. But you don't find it in a test tube. You can't buy a box of consciousness. If you could, chronic fatigue sufferers would be first in line, buying some on their way to work. So, eventually, even something as abstract as quantum physics has to turn its gaze on the even more abstract field of consciousness, in order to account for all known phenomena.

But the fact that quantum physicists are starting to investigate and speculate about consciousness doesn't mean that the emergency room at Parkview Central has been immediately affected. Most of modern medicine is based on an older model of physics, where billiard-ball atoms bond or bounce off of each other to make up our world. What this means is that even though the newest theories in Western science are beginning to glimpse what may be some universal perspectives that will radically alter our world view, practical medicine based on that world view is years away. Or maybe decades away.

Unless of course, we go straight to Maharishi Vedic Medicine, which was designed from the ground up (a long, long time ago) using the consciousness-as-primary model.

What if it was our connection to consciousness that determined how healthy we were, not the other way around? What if consciousness were a kind of primary field which was expressed in physical phenomena, or in our case, in mental and physical aspects of our lives?

The "what if" is now supported by research studies that indicate that experiences of fundamentally different states of consciousness are within the range of contemporary human experience, and that these states can be shown to have profound effects on individual physiology, psychology, and behavior.

As stated above, scientific research has shown an intimate connection between mind and body, such that particular states of consciousness have easily identifiable physiological correlates in the body. Similarly, over 400 research studies on the Transcendental Meditation Program (TM), one of the modalities of Maharishi Vedic Medicine, have shown that TM practitioners experience a unique state of consciousness during the practice. This state of consciousness is evidently worthy of detailed consideration, in comparison to the other states of consciousness that we normally experience.

The studies on the Transcendental Meditation Program indicate that during the practice there is a significant drop in respiration rate and blood lactate levels, and increased skin resistance all indicative of a deep state of rest.[4] Other research shows increased use of brain reserves during the practice,[5] as if more of the brain is activated, and that activation takes place in both hemispheres of the brain at the same time, indicating a more unified style of mental functioning.

All this indicates that the individual practicing the Transcendental Meditation Program is experiencing a deep state of rest, but that it is not an experience of the dullness of deep sleep, but a hypometabolic, highly integrated state of restful alertness. In practical terms, you are deeply rested but also more "together," in a calm, simple, unified,

---

4. Dillbeck MC, Orme-Johnson DW. Physiological differences between Transcendental Meditation and rest. *American Psychologist* 1987 42(9):879-881

5. Human Physiology 25: 171-180, 1999

peaceful state that both rejuvenates and energizes.

The studies indicate that the Transcendental Meditation program brings profound rest to the body, alertness on the part of the mind, and that these experiences affect both mind and body in a positive way, and that those effects continue into daily activity.

This experience, which has been repeated by millions of people in the last 50 years, all over the globe, has opened the door for improving psychological and physiological abnormalities, by exposing people to enhanced experiences of consciousness itself. This, the infusion of more consciousness into your life and your physiology through the Transcendental Mediation Program and many other related modalities, is the focus and basis of Maharishi Vedic medicine.

Your Perfect, Intelligent Body

Looking at your body from the perspective of consciousness is completely backward from what normally happens in the doctor's office. Here, in this book, instead of talking about you as if you are sick, we are going to talk about you in terms of what Maharishi Vedic Medicine considers your true nature: a perfectly functioning, intelligent being.

We're going to start with a perfectly healthy, highly conscious individual (you) and in the next chapters see how things may have become clouded over time to change that beautiful creation into a fatigued remnant of its former glory.

So let's continue discussing pure consciousness, which, even though we have started to talk about it, is perhaps as abstract to your experience as anything could be, and also, as far removed from fatigue as possible.

This discussion can get rather abstract, but please stay with it, since the payoff is enormously valuable for your health.

First of all, Maharishi Vedic Science looks at the primordial level of both microscopic (individual) and macroscopic (cosmic) existence as a field of energy and intelligence, or pure consciousness. Since this field is not bounded in time or space, it could be said to be an unbounded field, which, since we are talking about energy and intelligence, means that it is a field of unlimited energy. Which is a lot. More energy than you've been having recently, for one thing.

Let's imagine a field of unlimited, pure consciousness, energy and intelligence. Let's assume that it is completely alone, undifferentiated. No creation to think about. Just consciousness. A pure field of unlimited energy and intelligence, without any form or matter around it, no universe, no solar systems, no planets, no New Jersey.

So what does it do? Consciousness, by its own nature, seeks something to be conscious of, and so this pure field of consciousness naturally is drawn to become conscious of the only thing it can find....itself.

So, pure consciousness, without really losing its true nature as pure consciousness takes on the role of being the observer and the observed. And, we can note at this point, that if there is an observer and an observed, there can also be seen to exist a process of observation.

The ancient tradition of knowledge on which MVM is based is written primarily in Sanskrit, which has terms for these three aspects of consciousness; rishi (observer), devata (process of observation) and chandas (observed). The important thing to remember here is that these are simply roles or appearances of differentiation of the basic field of pure consciousness. They give the appearance of separation, while of course nothing has really changed on the level of pure consciousness.

What this means is that the original pure consciousness has become a three part thing, and yet it continues to be a wholeness of its own. It is both three and one at the same time. There is a kind of breaking of the infinite symmetry of one unified field into the diversity of three elements, and then a kind of reunification of the three back into one. This dynamic relationship of one into three and three into one is said to be the foundation for the dynamic, energetic aspect of pure consciousness.

Of course, once you have (apparently) three actors on stage, they can (appear to) interact with each other in various ways, as if a number of basic elements were combining. Out of these combinations, a whole world of apparent realities starts to get generated. It doesn't take long before the drama of the apparent realities starts to be taken seriously and the connection to the original substance, pure consciousness, is forgotten.

This is called the "mistake of the intellect," or pragyaparadh, i.e. when consciousness becomes forgetful of its true nature as the primordial, unified, unbounded, eternal field.

This may not sound like a big deal to practical existence but the end result of that loss of connection can mean that nice people like us feel sick and tired all of the time. If we were able to maintain a more enlightened perspective we would automatically maintain an awareness of pure consciousness along with the increasing complexities, but the tendency is to get lost in the boundaries and differences and losing the wholeness.

The details of Maharishi Vedic Medicine are succinctly described in many ancient texts of what is known as "Ayurveda," the classical health system of ancient India. Classical texts on Ayurveda take this loss of connection to pure consciousness very seriously. Thus far we have been discussing this disconnection from a purely abstract, cosmic perspective. But the disconnection of the individual from pure consciousness can be said to parallel the cosmic perspective, and the results of that disconnection are said to be known by the following bad actions of the individual:

- Overstimulating natural urges (e.g. Eating)
- Suppressing natural urges (such as sleep, elimination, etc.)
- Overexertion
- Too much sexual intercourse
- Over use, under use, or untimely use of medical treatments
- Loss of modesty and good behavior
- Disrespect for respectable people

- Use of mentally deranging substances (drugs, alcohol, etc.)
- Actions taken at the wrong time and place (e.g. - staying up too late)
- Friendship with people who exhibit anti-social behavior
- Avoiding good behavior
- Bad actions taken due to envy, vanity, fear, anger, ignorance, intoxication and confusion.[6]

Good or bad, this process of differentiation or manifestation is nothing new to western science.[7] Modern science investigates the complicated process of manifestation of what physics calls "the unified field."

The scientists who have been investigating the effects of the experience of pure consciousness on practitioners of the Transcendental Meditation Program have come up with many parallels between the unified field as described in modern physics and the field of pure consciousness.

Without going into detail here, it is extremely likely that these apparently disparate fields of study are describing the same field of pure energy and intelligence, which lies at the basis of both individual consciousness and the entire physical creation as we know it. As a group of popular philosophers (the Beatles) said: "It's all one, don't you know?"

The theoretical investigations of modern physics has indicated that

---

6. Charaka Samhita, Sharirasthana 1. 102-108
7. H. Sharma and C. Clark, Contemporary Ayurveda
   (New York: Churchill Livingstone, 1998) pp. 9-13

the unified field manifests into five different "spin types" which give rise to the elementary particles that make up all of creation.

In the language of Maharishi Vedic Medicine, these spin types are seen to correspond to five basic forces or fields which have as their more concrete expression the five elements known as akasha (space), vayu (air), agni (fire), apu or jala (water), and prithivi (earth).

In discussing human physiology, MVM describes these elements as combining to form what are called doshas, vata dosha from space and air, pitta dosha from fire and water, and kapha dosha from water and earth. More on these three in Chapter 3.

The Five Mahabhutas

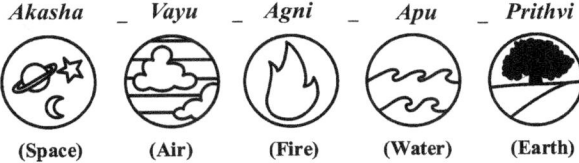

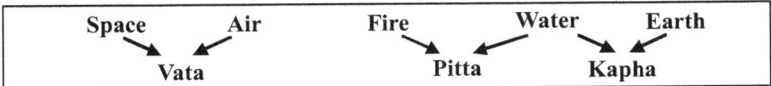

CHAPTER 3

Show Me the Dosha

Maharishi Vedic Medicine identifies the three organizing principles, vata, pitta , and kapha as they manifest in the human physiology. These dosha types are present in every human body, to varying degrees. The predominance of one or more doshas, therefore, is useful in defining individual differences in basic physiological makeup.

In addition, imbalances in the body can be identified in reference to imbalances in vata, pitta or kapha aspects of the physiology. It will be helpful, at this point, to identify some of the qualities of these three dosha types:

Vata: moving, quick, light, cold, rough, dry
Pitta: hot, sharp, light, acidic, slightly oily, liquid, flowing
Kapha: heavy, oily, slow, cold, steady, solid, dull, soft, sweet

The chart below gives a detailed description, along with the Ayurvedic names for each

Qualities of the three doshas:
Vata
- Ruksha - dry, rough
- Shita - cold, cool
- Laghu - light
- Sukshma - subtlety, minuteness
- Chala - movement

- Vishada - clarity, non-stickiness
- Khara - coarse, brittle

Pitta
- Sasneha - slight oiliness
- Ushna - heat, warmth
- Tikshna - sharp
- Drava - Liquid
- Amla - sour
- Sara - movement, flow
- Katu - pungent

Kapha
- Guru - heavy
- Shita - cold, cool
- Mridu - soft
- Snigdha - unctuous, oily
- Madhura - sweetness
- Sthira - stable, steady
- Picchila - stick, slimy
- Manda - dull, flat.[8]

According to Maharishi Vedic Medicine, these doshas have predominant functions in the body, vata governing transportation, movement and communication, pitta facilitating metabolism, digestion and transformation, and kapha contributing structure and cohesion.

They also are seen to have "seats" or predominant locations where they function in the body, since vata functions mainly in the colon, pitta in small intestine and stomach, and kapha in the chest.[9]

---

8. Charaka Samhita, Sharirasthana 1. 59-61
9. Charaka Samhita, Sutrasthanam 20. 8

Of course, it doesn't stop there, since there are five subdoshas of each dosha, and they all each have their favorite hangout in the body, too, but I won't go into that level of detail right now (more on this soon). The overview is that vata dosha relates to bodily movement of all kinds, pitta deals with digestion, and kapha handles little things like moistening and bodily structure.

These doshas aren't always bad boys. Normally they are in balance. When that happens with vata you have alertness, normal elimination, good sleep, strong immunity and can feel pretty much exhilarated. Good pitta means that you have normal body temperature, thirst and digestion, a sharp mind and a shiny complexion. Kapha can give strength, stamina, kindness, courage, mental stability and strong joints. All good things.

But when they go bad, look out, because vata imbalances leave you with rough skin, insomnia, constipation, fatigue (sound familiar?), headaches, anxiety, and mental imbalances, while pitta shows up with rashes, ulcers, heartburn, premature graying, balding, hostility and/or generally "going postal." Then kapha lumbers in with it's load of slow digestion, congestion, allergies, asthma, cysts, growths, and that big favorite, obesity.

But we're going to show you how to make those doshas behave.

One way these three express themselves (good or bad) is through their effects on the "dhatus" or tissues of the body.

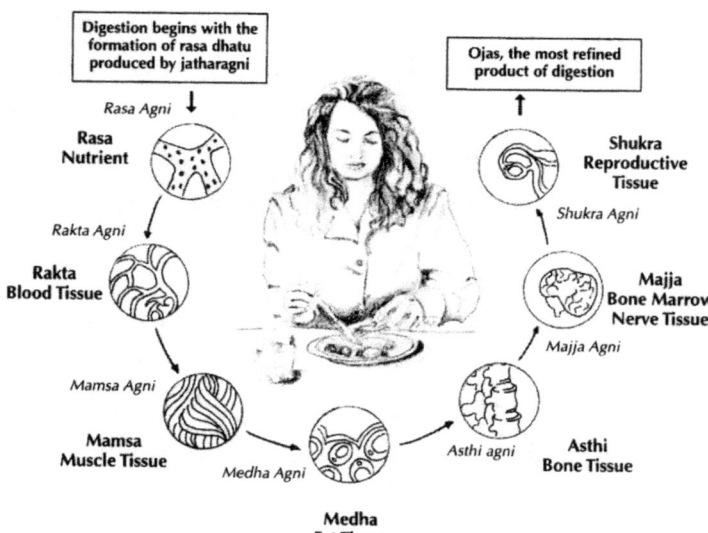

The Dhatu Construction Committee

Ayurvedic texts identify the following dhatus: rasa, rakta, mamsa, medha, ashti, majja, and shukra, which, in case your Sanskrit isn't that sharp right now (must be that fatigue). The first product of digestion is plasma (rasa), blood and hemoglobin (rakta), muscle (mamsa), fat (medha), bone (ashti), marrow and nervs (majja) and reproductive tissues (shukra).[10]

According to MVM, if these tissues are healthy and your doshas are in balance, you are healthy. Plus that little enlightened consciousness thing.

Sushrut Samhita (another ayurvedic text) has something to say about this:

---

10. Charaka Samhita, Chikitsasathanam 15. 15-17

Definition of a Healthy Individual:

"He whose doshas are in balance, whose appetite is good, whose dhatus are functioning normally, whose malas [see below] are in balance, and whose Self, mind and sense remain full of bliss, is called a healthy person."[11]

Of course, just because we can define health doesn't mean that we have it.

One reason for that is what that quote referred to as malas. Malas are the waste products created in forming the dhatus. If there are blockages in the physiology and these waste products can't eliminate properly, toxins accumulate. This throws off the natural, intelligent functioning of the body and imbalances result.

How the Dhatus Develop Sequentially to form Shukra Tissue	
Rasa ♦ Rakta ♦ Mamsa ♦ Meda ♦ Ashti ♦ Majja ♦ Shukra	
DHATUS	CORRESPONDING TISSUES
Rasa	Plasma, the first product of digestion and metabolism
Rakta	Blood, including hemoglobin
Mamsa	Muscle tissue
Meda	Fat tissue
Asthi	Bone tissue
Majja	Bone marrow, tissue of the nervous system
Shukra	Reproductive tissues

The sequential development of the dhatus					
Ojas ♦ Rasa ♦ Rakta ♦ Mamsa ♦ Meda ♦ Ashti ♦ Majja ♦ Shukra ♦ Ojas					
⇕	⇕	⇕	⇕	⇕	⇕
Ojas	Ojas	Ojas	Ojas	Ojas	Ojas

The aspects of the body that we have just presented, as described by

---

11. Sushruta Samhita Sutrasthanam 15. 38

29

Maharishi Vedic Medicine, are most of the players in the physiological drama that concerns us right now, i.e.- how we got sick and how to get "un-sick" again. However, there are a few crucial characters in the drama that we haven't yet met.

Three More Actors

Three more elements are worth introducing at this point in our health-related saga, and they are agni, ama and the srotas. Agni is the Vedic term for the elements in the body that have to do with digestion. Strong agni means strong digestion, or digestive "fire." There is a lot more to be said about agni (later), but for now it's enough to understand that MVM considers that there are types of agni associated with each dhatu, since MVM considers that each of the dhatus form the basis for developing the next dhatu in a specific sequence.

There is, therefore, a specific agni to transform rasa into rakta, and another specific form of agni to transform rakta into mamsa, etc. The agni that transforms rasa into rakta is called rasa agni; the agni changing rakta into mamsa is rakta agni, etc. The agni is said to "cook" the dhatu, producing the subsequent dhatu plus the malas or waste products of that process.

The following chart illustrates the process:

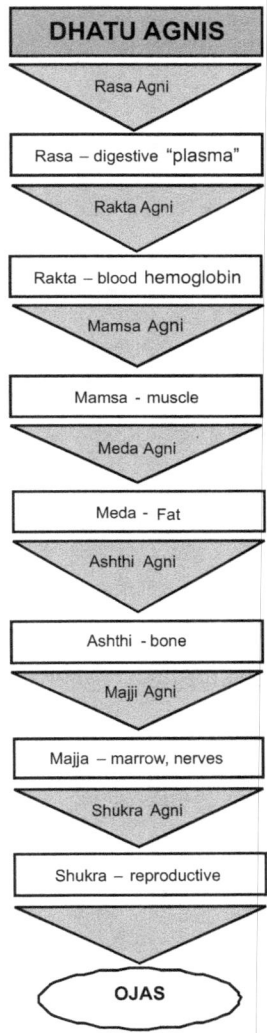

The quality of all of this transformation, however, is based on the quality of the basic form of agni, called jatharagni, which breaks down food products directly and forms the first dhatu, rasa or plasma. If jatharagni is balanced, it digests food properly, and all goes well with the dhatus, it is nourishing. If jatharagni is weak or too strong, or imbalanced in some other way, it produces poorly digested nutrients along with some well-digested nutrients. The poorly digested materials are called ama.

Ama is bad stuff. Sticky, icky, smell-bad stuff. If you were looking for the bad guy in this story, this is a chief candidate. Chronic fatigue is virtually indistinguishable from what is known as an "ama-condition" by Ayurvedic physicians. The body is just clogged up with gunk. This stuff slows down the functioning of the physiology and lowers physiological efficiency. And since it is full of impurities it can't get through the tiny pores in the body's tissues that allow physiological processes to flow smoothly.

Those "pores," or channels, are our third character, the srotas. The srotas are all of the channels in the body that connect the tissues. These can be large or small or any size between, since they include everything from nose and mouth down to tiny channels carrying nutrients to each cell. There are specific srotas for each dhatu.

When ama blocks the srotas, the functioning of the dosha and the agni in that area is compromised. Then the organ doesn't function properly, and it becomes a weak link in your overall heath. That weak link will prove to be important later in our drama, when the ama and the plot thickens.

The Doshas in Detail

Now let's look in detail at the various subtypes (five each) of each dosha, in order to see how each may have been part of how you become tired in the first place.

Looking at the five big vata types, we start out with prana vata, which means "vital breath," which is located in your head and chest, and includes heart, lungs, throat, tongue, mouth, and nose. Breathing polluted, stale, contaminated air or smoking could have contributed to problems in this arena.

Udana vata means "moving upwards," is located in the navel, chest and throat, and has to do with speech, singing, effort, energy, strength, and complexion. Blockages in this would sap energy.

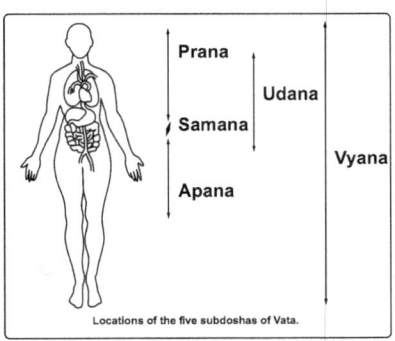

Locations of the five subdoshas of Vata.

Samana vata means "moving evenly" and is associated with sweat channels and digestive fire. It forms the fires of digestion. If you aren't digesting properly, your energy-producing machine isn't even getting a chance to turn over.

Apana vata means "moving downward," and governs organs of reproduction and elimination. This deals with many of the basic plumbing jobs: fecal elimination, urination, semen, menstrual blood, and delivering the fetus. You need smooth flow here to move out the old stuff. If you don't clear out the old, you start to feel it.

Vyana vata is "moving in all directions," and is located all over the body. It controls general movements of the body, extensions, contractions and circulation. Without freshness in this area you could be stiff and slowed.

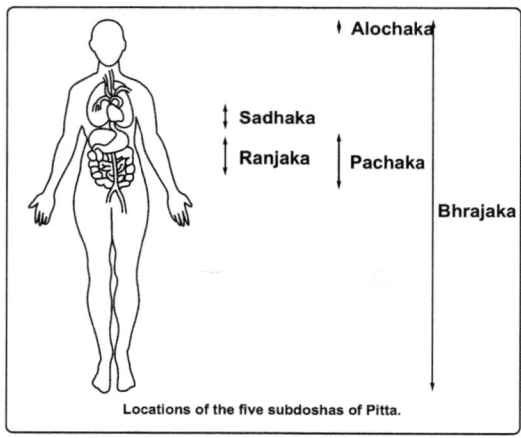

Locations of the five subdoshas of Pitta.

Pitta starts with pachaka pitta, which is a major player in the health game, since it means to "digest", "transform" or "cook". It does its work in the small intestine and duodenum and digests food and maintains the digestive fire. If you can't cook the food you can't "eat" the food-nutrients aren't getting in to stoke the fires, and you slow down to a halt.

Ranjaka pitta means "to color." It is in the liver and duodenum, and, since it forms and colors the blood, it governs all of the complex functions of the blood. You need good flow here. Maybe you've heard of "tired blood." You don't want that.

Sadhaka pitta means to "achieve" or "fulfill", it is associated with the heart, and governs little things like achieving desires, intelligence, intellectual acuity, memory, enthusiasm, ego, energy, and eliminating delusions. If you don't have this, you have no zest, no get up and go. Sound familiar?

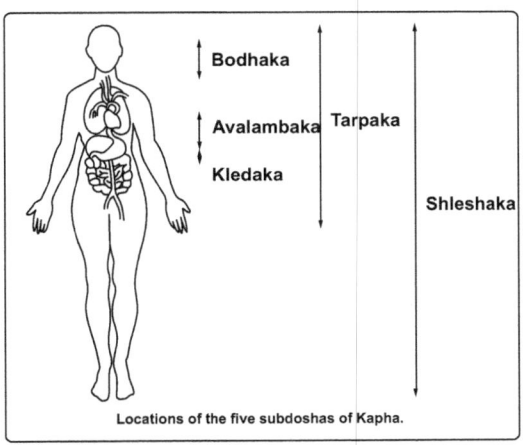

Locations of the five subdoshas of Kapha.

Alochaka pitta means "to see completely," rules the visual system including the visual cortex, and has to do with both outer and inner vision. In order to see the world as a brighter place, you have to "see" your true self (within), and in that light, re-view your life (without).

Pitta rounds out with bhrajaka pitta, which means "to light or shine," is associated with the skin, and controls the luster and shade of the skin, along with affecting the absorption of medicinal oils through the skin. Since the skin is the largest organ in the body, just purifying the skin can make a real difference.

Kapha kicks off with kledaka kapha ("to moisten"), which happens in the stomach and brings on the initial moistening and digestion of food. You need moisture or else your kapha turns into ama and you'll feel dull.

Avalambaka kapha means "double supporting" and functions in the chest, heart, and lower back in providing strong muscles, protecting the heart and keeping the chest, lungs and back strong. If you are feeling weak, this is probably affected.

Bodhaka kapha is associated with the tongue and throat in moistening the tongue, handling secretions of mucus membranes in the mouth, plus supporting the sense of taste. If you have lost your taste for life, this may be affected.

Tarpaka kapha means "pleasing" and "nourishing", and nourishes the mind, senses, spinal column and motor organs. If you are not receiving nourishment and pleasure from your food, it's not all in your head.

Shleshaka kapha means to "stick together", "bind" or "join". You hope this one is working because it has to do with lubrication of the joints and the general cohesion and/or binding of the whole body. If you are stiff and inflexible, (joint pain?), you might need work here.

That's the detailed view of all of your doshas. As you can see, problems in any one of these areas can potentially contribute to a chronically fatigued condition. And, if any one of them is imbalanced, that whole area is affected.

These doshas can be in balance (sama) or imbalanced in several ways, i.e. - by being too strong or too weak (termed "vitiated).

See the following chart for the details. The first one is the one you wish for:

Dosha State	Effect
Sama (balanced)	Health
Vriddhi (aggravated, increased)	Manifestation of signs/symptoms (depending on the degree of aggravation)
Kshina (diminished, decreased)	Absence of signs/symptoms

Let's say, however, that all of your doshas are in perfect running order (sama). That's great. But they still have to communicate with each other, and that takes place through the srotas.

Srotas in Detail

You'd be surprised at how many ways these srotas can go wrong. They can be blocked because they collapse. They can be blocked by ama. They can deteriorate. The stuff flowing through them can flow the wrong way. Stuff that's supposed to go both ways can be blocked from going one way. Stuff that's supposed to flow can just sit there. In any case, you need all these channels to be open and healthy.

And there's a bunch of them. You've got intake srotas for the respiratory system, srotas that which move the food aspect of the digestive system, and srotas which control water transport and metabolism. All of these channels must be functioning smoothly or you will have blockages that will slow you down.

Then there's a bunch of srotas that carry plasma, blood and lymph. If your tissues aren't getting nourished, you might feel a bit fatigued (sound familiar?) There's srotas that carry blood and hemoglobin, and that feed the muscles (weak muscles = feeling weak). Some types nourish the fat tissues, some supply the bones, or help out the bone marrow, nerve and brain tissue. All of those need to be strong, or you aren't. The male and female reproductive systems each have their own srotas. Cell membrames and cells have srotas as well.

There's also those hard-working waste removal srotas for feces and sweat. Constipation is almost an automatic cause of fatigue. When your bowels aren't moving you feel deadened and slowed. Smooth elimination, as basic as it is, can be a cause for elation.

On the other hand, assuming that all this machinery is going great, your dhatu/tissues are excellent, the communication via the srotas is clear, and all of your doshas and subdoshas are humming along just fine, thank-you, plus your diet, behavior and emotional life are in order, your body, according to MVM, is probably producing substantial amounts of a very fine substance called ojas (see dhatuagni chart, above).

Ojas is nothing but good news to the body. Ojas is said to be one of the finest aspects of individual existence, because it functions right there on the fine junction point between consciousness and matter.

It could be said to be the material counterpart or manifestation of the pure happiness or bliss aspect of pure consciousness. When ojas is lively in your physiology, it creates enthusiasm and a feeling of fulfillment on the level of the mind, and nourishment throughout the body. If you are low on ojas you feel emaciated, lazy, impotent and confused. Sound familiar?

Ojas has to do with "bala," a term which means mental and physical strength, but is usually used to mean resistance to disease, or simply health. Ojas keeps all of the variables of dosha, dhatu and agni functioning smoothly, and that means you just don't get sick.

Sushruta Samhita has nothing but nice things to say about ojas:

"The pure intelligence or essence of the dhatus, rasa, etc., ending with shukra, is called the auspicious ojas and also bala [strength, immunity] in the authentic text.

By bala or ojas, mamsa [muscle] becomes full, all movements become free and perfectly coordinated, voice and complexion become clear, and externally and internally the activity of the organs of action and the sense organs become self-referral, intelligent and evolutionary.

Ojas, which is of the nature of soma, is: snigdha (unctuous), shukla (white), shital (cool), sthira (stable), sara (moving/flowing), vivikta (pure in quality), mridu (soft), mritsna (cohesive), and is located at the very sprouting of life.

Being omnipresent in living beings, ojas nourishes every part of the body. Deficiency of ojas is equal to the destruction of the body of living beings."[12]

You can see that, from the perspective of MVM, a healthy body could be viewed as a finely tuned, ojas production machine. So, assuming that you have that perfect, ojas-saturated body, you would have a smoothly running engine composed of all of the elements we have discussed, and yet still be connected in a very real sense to that inner field of unlimited energy and intelligence from which it is truly constructed, that field of pure consciousness.

In that perfect state, your body is brimming with inner intelligence, there is perfect communication and coordination of all the parts, and since you are aware of all the levels of your existence all the way from your baby finger to the primordial level of pure consciousness, and the inner communication of information about what feels good, what foods are right to eat, and what behaviors are best in any one moment is pretty much automatic.

In addition, since there is so much internal coherence, the integrity of your system is much stronger than the entropic elements that surround you, and you are as if stronger than disease, so diseases just can't penetrate the invincible armor of your healthy system.

If this describes you, you are one healthy person. Of course, that perfect state may have been a while ago, or, more likely, strictly imaginary to most people. Let's see why…

---

12. Sushruta Samhita Sutrasthanam 15. 19-22

CHAPTER 4

The Bad News:
Rated PG-13 for Self-inflicted Violence

So, you had that really nice machine. Or something like it. But, since you didn't know much about machines, you did a few things wrong in the maintenance arena, little stuff, like you put in the wrong fuel, missed checkups, bought some bad spare parts, cheap paint, the wrong additives, neglected the timing, and put it in a bad garage, etc. And you still wonder why "the thing don't run like it used to."

Let's look at what you may have done slightly wrong in the maintenance of your perfect body.

Fuel

Your perfect body likes fresh vegetables and food that still has some life force in it. Freshly picked, just cooked food is best. But you have been feeding it containerized, highly processed food that last saw the light of day a year or so ago. They put an expiration date on the can, but, I'm sorry, that food was dead the day they canned it.

You've been eating processed food, lots of sugars, a bizarre combination of depressants and stimulants such as alcohol and caffeine, an occasional stray vitamin here and there, but no real balance or plan.

What if you are predominantly a vata body type, which flourishes under the influence of warm regular cooked meals, but you've been eating cold milk, ice cream, cookies and crackers on your occasional snack run through the employee vending machine area? I think we mentioned that vata is dry and cold. That means you've been making that dry, cold physiology drier and colder. Your body is already naturally leaning that way, but you thought you'd go for completely freeze-dried.

Or, you are a pitta-type and you love hot, spicy food, but never notice that you get angry and overheated afterwards. Pitta. Hot. "Uh… not need more fire." (It's that simple.)

Or maybe (surprise, surprise) you are mostly kapha but eat heavy foods with lots of sauces and gravy. As if you needed more ballast.

What we need to discuss here is the difference between samanya and vishesh. Samanya means "same," or "like." Eating something that has the same quality as your individual physiology will naturally increase that quality. Eating something that is vishesh to your basic physiological quality will decrease or cause diminution of that quality.

Charaka Samhita indicates that exposure, not just to food, but to herbs, treatments, environments or behaviors that are similar to your doshic condition will increase that quality. Conversely, exposure to any quality will also decrease (vishesh) the opposite quality, e.g. - exposure to dryness will decrease unctuousness in the body, softness will decrease hardness, etc.[13]

In all of the cases described above you are engaging in samanya type

---

13. Charaka Samhita, Sutrasthanam 1. 44-45

food behaviors, which are aggravating your basic condition. If you were still in touch with your body's inner intelligence--which by the way is always sending us messages, it's just that we have stopped listening--you wouldn't be eating that stuff. You might even be naturally discovering vishesh causing foods.

Bear in mind, that some times samanya foods might be used on purpose to increase a quality in your physiology, such as pitta (to improve digestion) or kapha (to bring peace to a busy mind).

At this point you are perhaps thinking that we're going to tell you that you would be better off becoming a total vegetarian. However, for some people it's actually too much of a shock to the system to make a total change like that right away. Especially due to the fact that such a completely different diet has to be carefully designed so that you get complete nutrients from new sources.

On the other hand, moving in that direction wouldn't be a bad idea, since, if you are what you eat (which is an extreme view, but it certainly gets attention), I might remind you that meat is clearly dead by definition, and if you eat the dead it may have, at least, a deadening effect. And anything that slows you and your digestion down is particularly suspect in the case of someone who is combating fatigue.

I could say a lot more about this, but you get the general drift. At least a move toward lighter meats like chicken and fish is in order (depending on your dosha type) and maybe go for the whole thing if and when it makes sense for you.

If you've been putting bad fuel in (and who hasn't?) you have been making jatharagni's job very difficult, and so you are not helping maintain that perfect body. The body may have started out okay, but if you have a child and then feed the child a breakfast made out of oatmeal and sugar, you probably aren't going to end up with a healthy kid. And that's not much different than what you've been shoving into the equation.

In the computer programming world they have an acronym, G.I.G.O., which stands for "garbage in, garbage out," meaning that if you put in poor programming information, you are going to get out poor data. The same is true of the body.

The problem is that we don't normally think of the body as producing anything. But now that we have learned that the body is not only always producing itself, as one dhatu becomes the basis for the next, but also the magic stuff called ojas as the end product, we understand how crucial it is that we provide high quality raw (or cooked) materials for this process to have any hope of succeeding.

On the other hand, from the perspective of Maharishi Vedic Medicine, a truly healthy physiology could make ojas out of almost any food, within reason. But most of us are far from such perfect health, so when you put bad food in, your body labors mightily, but it just can't make silky ojas out of a sow's cold, leftover ham. So what happens is that poor food, poorly digested, becomes the input to your tissue development process, and that results in that gloppy, sticky ama stuff becoming part of what you are feeding yourself internally, part of the general rasa dhatu, part of the rakta dhatu, mamsa dhatu, etc. In that case you have started to cloud and srota-block the functioning of that perfect body you started out with.

As you will see from the information extracted from Charaka Samhita below, food behaviors dominate the list of what's bad for the srotas (channels) and agni (digestive fire). You may see some things that you have experienced or done now and then on the list. If not, you are one lucky human!

Factors Vitiating Srotas

In general, srotas may be vitiated by:

- Overeating
- Eating before your previous meal is digested (e.g. eating snacks between meals)
- Unwholesome food. Food or drink that is clearly bad for you alcohol, stale food, etc.
- Incompatible food (incompatible with your physiology)
- Incompatible food (creating poor food combinations)
- Sleeping after meals
- Too much exercise
- Too little exercise
- Weak digestion
- Suppressing natural urges (see below)
- Too much heat or cold
- Concussion or Shock
- Excessive worries

Basically, foods and behaviors that are bad for the doshas and dhatus are also bad for the srotas.[14]

Factors Deranging Agni

- Fasting
- Over-eating
- Eating before your previous meal is digested
- Irregular eating
- Eating during indigestion
- Eating bad food
- Suppressing natural urges
- Wrong use of enemas
- Emaciation due to some disease
- Problems adapting to changes of location, climate, and season
- Experiencing anger, worries, and sorrow [15]

Survival can probably be accomplished, for a while, with substandard food. But perfect health, realization of your highest potential, cannot.

When we look at life as containing the possibility of enlightenment, as having within reach a state of perfect health where our mind and body are totally in tune with the inner intelligence of nature, where we have perfect health on the level of the body, and perfect, exalted, energetic, totally free and unlimited potential as our second-by-second experience on the levels of the mind and inner self, we suddenly acquire a higher goal for our existence than simple survival.

---

14. Charaka Samhita, Vimanasthana 5. 23

15. Charaka Samhita, Chikitsasathanam 15. 42-44

And it's nothing other than what you really are. At least what we decided you were in the last chapter. It's just that pragyaparadh, the mistake of the intellect, has come into full force, and you have "forgotten" your full nature. Maharishi Vedic Science, therefore, is simply here to enliven your memory, called smriti, of your true nature.

On the other hand there are a few things you've been doing that your body would like to forget, like the alcohol that you have consumed, or the cigarettes that you've been smoking. Maybe your race car runs on pure alcohol, but your body doesn't, since it has an incredibly dulling and neuron-killing effect on your organic machine. Plus your air intake system doesn't work best when it is burnt and tarred over by cigarette smoke.

Timing

Then there's that little problem with your timing:

It turns out that the body has cycles of functioning, daily, circadian cycles, as well as cycles of adjustment to varying seasons. Maharishi Vedic Medicine has indicated that the three dosha types also hold sway over times of the day, vata being most dominant in the hours of 2-6 (both a.m. and p.m.), kapha from 6 to 10, and pitta from 10 to 2.

What that means, for example, is that it's best to arise in the morning before 6 a.m., while nature is light and lively with the vata influence. After 6 a.m., the heaviness of kapha sets in and dullness of mind and body are the inevitable result (for dullness read: ama). Similarly, it's great for the body if you go to bed before 10, because the slowness of the evening hours is conducive to deeper sleep, while if you stay up past 10, the more lively energy of pitta isn't as supportive of falling deeply asleep.

The mid-day pitta hours are said to be the best time to eat the heaviest meal of the day, because that's when digestion is the strongest. Of course, many people eat a big meal at night, in the middle of the slowest digestive time. A good portion of that slowly digesting food becomes hardly digested food once you fall asleep, and then it ends up as more of your questionable physiological associate, ama.

The pitta hours of 10 p.m. to 2 a.m. are considered to be a good time for pitta to "burn off" the impurities collected in the body during the day, as part of the sleep cycle, but if you instead occupy the body with extra digestion, or if you don't rest the body at that time anyway, that fine, intelligent capability of the body never engages properly, and stress and impurities inexorably accumulate.

Flowing with changes in climate and geography are also important, since when a dosha increases in the environment, it also increases in our bodies. MVM describes a number of things we can do to balance the doshas when the seasons change, such as changes in diet, herbs, exercise levels, dress, etc. This seasonal routine is called ritucharya. For instance, in the summer, when the weather warms up, pitta increases in our bodies as well as in the environment, and MVM naturally recommends a pitta-pacifying diet.

Driving Habits

Ayurveda also identifies several major sources of imbalance and disease with reference to mental, physical and speech activity, and mistakes with reference to sensory experience.

Mental, physical, or speech activities can be inappropriate due to too much activity, not enough activity, or by the damaging content of the activity. Examples of too much activity would be talking too much; too much mental focus or pressure; improper exercise or over-exertion; too much traveling; or consistently irregular routine. Not enough activity would appear in not speaking much or keeping silent for long periods; mental idleness or laziness; physical inertia or laziness; insufficient exercise; suppressing natural urges and functions (coughing, sneezing, urinating, etc.). "Damaging content" examples in the speech arena would be lying, gossip, harsh and abusive speech; irrelevant speech; or speech which focuses on others' faults. Mental mistakes would be fear, anger, greed, and other toxic emotions. Physical imbalance results from, among other things, sleeping on uneven places and activity which endangers life, such as physical assault, alcohol and drug use, fire, exposure to radiation or toxic environments.

Certain emotions can cause imbalances or exacerbate existing ones, just as wrong food does. Vata is aggravated by fear, grief, anxiety, pressure and stress. Pitta is aggravated by anger, irritability, over-excitement, emotional intensity, and competitiveness. Kapha is aggravated by passion, greed, attachment and jealousy.

Misuse of the senses is also problematic, since taking information and stimuli into our minds and bodies through our senses is considered to be similar to eating. If the content of experience is inappropriate, excessive or over-stimulating, under-stimulating, or harsh, destructive, or toxic in nature the result can be the formation of mental and emotional ama, which impairs mental and emotional functioning and ultimately can cause disease.

For instance, after we hear sad or frightening news, we may keep thinking about it all day and have trouble focusing on work. Waves of anxiety may come and go throughout the day. We might also have difficulty falling asleep, or our sleep is restless and disturbed by emotional or violent dreams. Consequently, we feel physically tired in the morning and mentally sad or agitated, which in turn affects everything we do all day.

Steering

This is where the concept of pragyaparadh makes a difference. If we are deeply enmeshed in a distorted, one-sided view of life, i.e. - a view which doesn't include the infinite inner freedom of pure consciousness, where we have become stuck in the field of limitations and change without reference to our true nature, certain behavioral abnormalities become more likely.

It's easy to see why this would happen. It's unlikely that a millionaire would become a thief, just because the millionaire has so much already-what would a few more stolen dollars do? But if he has forgotten his riches, he may sink to lower levels of behavior.

A distorted view of one's self worth results in a distorted view of the environment, and, ultimately, wrong behavior based on those views. When you are not at ease with yourself, you tend to be ill at ease with others and, eventually, you begin to engage in some of the destructive behaviors described by Ayurvedic texts: undue desires, greed, pride, delusion or attachment, and jealousy.

We act wrong, we eat wrong, we go wrong. It's automatic. We normally restrain ourselves from illegal behaviors due to a combination of internal moral and external legal codes. But maybe by engaging in behavioral imbalances that are not in themselves strictly illegal or immoral, we still are in violation of other, natural laws. And that, due to such violations, we are somehow imprisoned in unhappiness and disease as a result, walled off and separated from true living.

There may be several levels of mistake of the intellect: feeling a separation of mind and body, or separation of intellect, emotions, body, and environment. This separated feeling has long since gripped the personal experiences and even philosophies of modern life. And any time we are not intrinsically aware that each of these components are expressions of infinite intelligence, on an experiential level, we are in the grip of an aspect of pragyaparadh. Which includes most of us.

The Garage

What about the garage you've been storing your (physiological) car in? Perhaps you've heard of "sick building syndrome." What that means to most people is that dust, asbestos, pollen and other contaminants are accumulating in buildings with little or no ventilation, and it's not hard to get sick in a building that sick.

But Maharishi Vedic Science takes that understanding to an even deeper level, through the knowledge of Maharishi Sthapatyaved, which is the science of designing the correct structure and orientation of buildings so that there is a positive effect on the inhabitants. I'll talk more on this topic later, but for now you can rest assured if you are living or working in a poorly ventilated building with plastic insulation and a southern entrance on the south slope of a hill overlooking a lake, you might as well go jump in that lake (and swim to the other side and start building).

The point of all this is that although we come out of the factory with some pretty fantastic machinery that actually has far more capabilities than we ever suspected, through lack of knowledge, guidance or inspiration we have slowly been destroying the machine.

It's as if a group of people from an aboriginal culture were given a jet plane, and yet were never instructed as to what the plane could do, and so they have taken to hanging the wash on the wings, towing it here and there, using it to float down river, sometimes as a percussion instrument, plus storing food in the engines, chipping off little pieces for jewelry, etc.

All interesting uses, of course, but wouldn't you rather fly in your beautiful machine? I suggest you take it into the shop for a diagnosis and a tune-up, and get a little preflight training/knowledge at the same time. Part of that knowledge is to understand what happened as a result of our improper behaviors, exactly what happens when you get sick. We'll unfold that drama in the next chapter.

But first a few more behaviors that may have contributed to imbalances that resulted in some serious fatigue. You may see some items that you recognize on the list:

Factors Aggravating the Three Doshas

Vata

- Staying awake too much at night, missing sleep
- Fear, grief, worry, anxiety, agitation, anger
- Excessive mental or physical work, exercise, too much travelling, speaking, strain and/or fatigue
- Suppressing natural bodily functions [see below]
- Fasting (in some cases), not eating enough food
- Eating too much vata type foods: rough, dry, light, astringent and bitter foods
- Wasting away, excessive weight loss (including loss due to fatigue)
- Vata "timing" elements, i.e., the effects of old age, early morning, late afternoon, dry, cold, windy and changing climates

- Irregular in daily and seasonal routines
- Injuries from falling down, e.g. bone fractures

Pitta

- Excessive exertion, speaking and thinking
- Exposure to too much heat and sunshine; a burning sensation and/or acidity in the body
- Experiences of anger, hatred, jealousy, passion
- Fasting (sometimes)
- Eating pitta foods: hot, sharp, sour, salty and pungent foods
- Using alcohol and smoking tobacco
- Pitta "timing" (middle age, midday, midnight, hot weather)

Kapha

- Too much rest and sleep (sleeping in the daytime, after meals, etc.), Not enough exercise and/or mental and physical work
- Eating too much
- Kapha food, i.e. - heavy, unctuous, cold, sweet, sour, saline, and also slimy and sticky food
- Kapha time (childhood, morning, evening, cold and wet climates)

Most of us have done one or two of those, which have contributed to our health problems. On the other hand, according to Charaka Samhita, there are a number of behaviors that you shouldn't repress, due to the blockages caused by restricting them, e.g. - urination, defecation, seminal discharge, flatulence, vomiting, sneezing, belching, yawning, hunger, thirst, tears, sleep and the heavier breathing caused by exertion.[16]

So, you can let all that go in the future. But we still may have to face what happened to us due to holding back in the past.

Most of what we have done wrong has weakened our constitution to the point where we are more likely to become ill. In the next chapter we'll look at the whole course of illness from the opening act to the final curtain. Hopefully your illness won't go the distance, but we have to have a sense of how the plot thickens before we can rewrite your tired story with a happy ending.

---

16. Charaka Samhita, Sutrasthanam 7. 3-4

CHAPTER 5

How You Got Sick, A Drama in Six Acts

Prologue

Of course, we'd like to prevent this kind of drama from starting at all. The Ayurvedic maxim is "heyam duhkham anagatam," or "avert the danger that has not yet come." Prevention is far more powerful than cure. In addition, handling a disease at any of the earlier stages of it's unfolding story (as described below) is easier than in the later stages. But in the case of most of us, it's a little too late for that, at least for some illnesses. Even so, we can learn how to prevent further damage, and how to keep such dramas from getting started in the future.

Most theatrical dramas take only three acts, and the story of a patient's sickness only has two acts, to most doctors: 1) they get sick and 2) we deal with it. But Maharishi Vedic Medicine identifies four stages that the illness went through before it even showed up for tryouts, which makes six acts in all.

Maybe you'd like to hear the whole story.

Act One

The first act is called Sanchaya, which means accumulation. When doshas get imbalanced, they usually increase. During Sanchaya, the doshas start to increase in their primary site, which for vata is the colon, kapha in the lungs, and pitta in the stomach and small intestine.

Even though the patient is far from what we would normally call sick at this stage, there may already be symptoms, for example with pitta sanchaya a slight increase in body temperature, and with kapha sanchaya a feeling of heaviness in the body.

Let's say that our two characters are named Tard (who is tired) and Sikntard (who is sick and tired). I'm going to give away the ending by telling you that Tard will end up with chronic fatigue by the end of the drama, while Sikntard will end up with Chronic Fatigue Syndrome.

Let's say that (Ms.) Tard starts to stay up late a lot, has a lot of demands placed on her, lots of changes. Her life becomes more and more vata-aggravating, and here in Act One she starts to accumulate excess vata in her colon. She might begin having mild constipation and gas effects, and her mental agitation would begin to exceed the degree and duration that is truly necessary to handle the problems that she faces. It's as if she begins to be in a constantly "up," emergency state mentally, and sleep begins to be a bit fitful and late in arriving.

Mr. Sikntard has the opposite problem. He eats too much, and too often. He doesn't exercise. Stays indoors most of the time. No fresh air, no friends. His digestion is slow, and yet he eats clogging foods (probably peanut butter, mixed with chocolate) that exceed the degree to which he can digest them efficiently. He starts to build up kapha in his lungs, maybe starting up a bit of a cold. At the least he begins to feel heaviness and "lassitude" - an educated word for "the slows."

In both of these cases, sites that house the specific doshas in the body (vata colon, kapha lungs) have started to show symptoms of imbalance.

Act Two

Usually the first act leads to the second, which is Prakopa, or spreading to other sites, plus an increase in severity. These sites are the subordinate sites associated with each dosha, as described earlier in this book. In this stage Ms. Tard may experience prickly pain in the alimentary tract, minor diarrhea, etc., in other words, areas other than the colon itself are starting to get affected. Mr. Sikntard may start to get an aversion to food or even nausea. And that cold gets worse, starting to congest the head.

Act Three

At this point these two will probably know that something is wrong, but without really knowing what to do about it, it may easily progress to the next phase, which is Prasara, or "spreading to a wider area." If the dosha imbalances are not controlled or eliminated in the second stage, the imbalances not only increase even more, they start spreading to the seats of the other doshas. So a pitta imbalance can start to affect other parts of the body than would normally be affected by pitta imbalances.

In the case of Tard, she may now be experiencing dry skin,

constipation, tension headaches, and more anxiety along with more things to be anxious about. Plus she may have gurgling noises in the alimentary tract, belching, all signs of processes moving the wrong way in the body's srotas. Sikntard, meanwhile, may be blessed with loss of appetite, loss of taste, indigestion, overall weakness of the body, and even vomiting.

Things are getting pretty mixed up at this point, and it is about here, where the internal drama of illness starts to get people's attention and they start thinking about going to a doctor, or at least to a pharmacy for some over-the-counter relief.

There's no shortage of Ayurvedic words to describe the many potential symptoms that can be noticed at this stage: nidranasa (loss of sleep), balopaghata (loss of strength), sukhopagata (loss of happiness), shoka (grief), manda-chesta (slow activity), apraharsha (not interested in anything), mudhasamjnata (slow intellect), kaphavriddhi (loss of appetite), balanasa (loss of strength), atripti (discontentment), apakti (indigestion) and alasya (lassitude).[17]

Bad news by any name.

Act Four

As wiped out as these people are, they still have to sit through Act Four (and remember, they're not even sick yet, if they ask their doctor). Act Four is called Sthana, or localization. At this point the dosha imbalances increase even further and start to interact with

---

17. K. R. S. Murthy, Doctrines of Pathology in Ayurveda,
    (Delhi, Chaukhambra Orientalia, Vidyavilas Ayurveda Series, No. 3, pp. 101-103

existing problem areas in your body that have already been weakened due to the ama/srota blockages that we described above, and major problems start to manifest in those specific locations.

It's as if a gang of rogue dosha imbalances has been roaming around the patient's body, jumping fences and looking for trouble, when they run smack into some grumpy ama-blocked srota tissues, and when those two forces tangle, some kind of street fight is certain to happen, with your body as the battleground. Sadly, of course, it's not really a meeting of powerful forces, but a gathering of weak, confused, and troubled elements, but even so, they can cause a lot more damage than a little rumble in the stomach.

What comes out of all this is what is called prodromal symptoms, the premonitions of illness, which in Sanskrit are called purvarupa. These include general symptoms of illness and specific symptoms which start to act like specific diseases, but in a subtle way that is hard to recognize.

Tard and Sikntard are probably still engaging in the activities that got them in this condition in the first place, so what's to keep these imbalances from increasing? So symptoms that may give a hint as to the nature of emerging, future diseases start to appear.

Act Five

All this sets the stage for the fifth act, the vyakti or manifestation section, where the imbalances get aggravated further and the patient has an obvious "roga" (i.e. - a disease, with all of it's clear symptoms).

At this point our two sickos take a different path. Of course, they are already on different paths due to their quite different physiologies, but something happens at this point to distinguish the two. Tard shows symptoms of chronic fatigue. But Sikntard, let's say, gets the flu, but never seems to recover. For some reason (as yet undetermined, remember), some people end up chronically fatigued, while others get CFS.

Chronic Fatigue is certainly serious, and needs treatment, but CFS is a far more serious condition. In any case, it's at this point in the outbreak phase where the differences between the two start to be obvious. Tard is tired, beat, dragging around, but Sikntard is both sick and tired, beat, exhausted, sure, but also with fevers, extreme weakness, no energy, little ability to exercise, etc.

Even so, now the villain is clearly visible onstage and even traditional medicine will commit itself to saying, "Hey, you're sick." It's at this point that the dramatic tricks of conventional medicine normally step in and it is business as usual, if that's the only kind of story that you know.

On the other hand, we could also start using Maharishi Vedic Medicine to retrace the origin and course of the disease, clearly determining which dosha is imbalanced, which area of the srotas is blocked, and start to undo the damage that has been caused. Which is a good thing, even if the patient has waited until Act Five to take action.

At this point, right in the middle of the fifth act, it's time for an intermission. Maybe it's a bit late in the show for an intermission, and normally we'd at least wait until the act is over, but we're already doing things differently than you're used to, so why stop now?

The reason for this break is that Maharishi Vedic Medicine brings out a new insight, which may shed light on Sikntard's problem: that elusive villain, Chronic Fatigue Syndrome. Maharishi Vedic Medicine can detect the imbalances even in the earlier stages before the manifestation of symptoms.

So let's take a break from the action and discuss this development in the lobby.

Intermission - Out In the Lobby:

Maharishi Vedic Medicine, identifies two kinds of dosha imbalances, which I will call Type G and Type S (not their real names, but you won't remember them anyway, so this is simpler). Type G imbalances are those that are increased by unsuitable personal activities and foods (see leftover ham, mentioned earlier), processed, packaged, preserved foods, and these imbalances circulate all over the body, producing general symptoms of illness. We described those activities in some detail in the last chapter.

The production of Type S imbalances are more likely to be caused by the combination of abnormally developed doshas with poorly functioning dhatus, with some ama and malas (waste products) thrown into the mix. Type S conditions produce symptoms that are more characteristic of specific diseases.

Type G, the general cause, has more symptoms and its manifestations are all over the body. The Type S aspect is considered less powerful, and it's effects are usually confined to specific areas. In Maharishi Vedic Medicine it is considered more important to treat the Type G aspect first, because it is the most powerful imbalance, and having done that, the Type S conditions will often disappear by themselves. In other words, in terms of the body, if you have healthy soil, the weeds can't sprout.

Having said all that, it's important to step back and see what this view of disease means, since it has major implications for both how we do medicine in general and our consideration of fatigue.

Like what? Like maybe traditional medicine can't see the forest for the trees. It would be considered superficial, even in traditional medicine, to simply treat the symptoms of an illness, rather than try to effect a cure. But it may turn out that particular illnesses are symptoms of a more general imbalance or illness that is creating a foundation on which specific illnesses are flourishing. That is certainly the perspective of Maharishi Vedic Medicine.

This would mean that the discovery of a specific illness, while delightful in some ways to the traditional medical practitioner, since he or she can now at least go to work, might also obscure the more fundamental origins and more profound cures potentially available to a doctor trained in Maharishi Vedic Medicine. What we usually do about illnesses may be like chopping off the top of a weed without rooting out what's below the ground. More problems surface soon thereafter.

It may also be possible that there are some diseases which are largely or even completely Type G based, with powerful symptoms noticed all over the body, but without much in the way of Type S symptoms. In this case, the patient would have all kinds of symptoms, but none of them could be traced to a particular illness. For example, a patient

- Could have:
- Mild fever
- Sore throat
- Painful lymph nodes
- Muscle weakness
- Muscle pain
- Prolonged fatigue after exercise
- Headaches
- Joint pain
- Neuropsychologic complaints
- Sleep disturbance
- Acute onset of symptoms
- Low grade fever
- Throat inflammation
- Palpable or tender lymph nodes

You may recall that list from Chapter 2. In other words, there may be illnesses, such as Chronic Fatigue Syndrome, which just don't show up on any of your doctor's tests for specific diseases, and yet you are really sick.

As a matter of fact, the very existence of a disease such as Chronic Fatigue Syndrome calls into question our traditional model of illness, because, according to the traditional model, there isn't any illness. If the model says you aren't sick, and you still have that list of symptoms, either you're crazy, or the model is wrong. Many people, of course, would prefer that you just agree to be considered crazy rather than adjust the nice model.

However, the Maharishi Vedic Medicine model may actually account for the mystery of the missing CFS diagnosis. You are sick all over, but you don't have a particular sickness. The ground state of your health is unsettled, but there's no sprouting up of anything that is verifiably based on a testable, traditional disease.

Any scientist worth his salt would typically be delighted by a theory which accounts for more of the observed phenomena, as this one does. We can of course ignore the apparent paradox of CFS and continue in our normal medical ways. But we are naturally attracted to a medical solution that both accounts more effectively for CFS and brings with it a wealth of effective cure modalities based on that wider view, i.e. - Maharishi Vedic Medicine.

This perspective may even allay the current frenzied search for a cause of Chronic Fatigue Syndrome. It may be that the specific quality of CFS is determined or influenced by some elusive causal factor, but the overarching problem may not be the triggering factor, but the general manifestations of illness due to long-standing doshic imbalances.

From the perspective of a Maharishi Vedic Medicine physician, most chronically fatigued patients, however they got that way, are suffering from an "ama condition." What that means is that an extreme buildup of poorly digested tissues or ama has built up in the body.

It may have happened due to a lack of digestive fire, since the digestion couldn't process food properly and you ended up with ama. It may have happened due to blockages in the srotas and wastes built up and you ended up full of ama. Or maybe your pitta was too high and your physiology overcooks everything and you get burnt tissues, which results in ama.

The point is that regardless of how you got there, the ama must be eliminated. The Maharishi Vedic Physician needs to take account of your particular physiology in order to eliminate the ama from your particular physiology more effectively and smoothly, but may not have to know the minutiae of how you got that way.

A myriad of causes, behavioral, dietary and environmental may have pushed you there. The road that you took on your descent into ill health may actually be perfectly clear to the MVM physician, but that's not as important as finding the road up out of the dark valley. Cause may not be as important as cure. The ama must go, and your physiological health and immunity must be built up from the inside out, in a way that is suited to you and you alone.

It is at this point that we would suggest you might go ahead and have one of those "aha" experiences, since we have just uncovered what may be the central point of this entire book, and also have provided what may be the master key for treating both Chronic Fatigue and CFS.

The point, in case it slipped by with all the traffic and other conversations going on out here in the lobby, is that by treating the underlying imbalance, we can take the energy out of the symptoms of your illness. Your illness is flourishing, evidently, on a deep bed of unrest. Your generalized sickness is allowing a number of symptoms to take root. If we treat the symptoms, we haven't eliminated the tradition of illness from your body… more problems can always spring up. If we eliminate the fundamental underlying malaise, the symptoms should lose force and diminish.

By turning this master key, we open the window to health for your entire physiology, and all those rascally little symptoms will not have anywhere to hide in the new, sunlit room that your body will become. But that's part of the happy sequel to the current tragedy, the one where things went bad in the first place.

Still, it may be that the most dramatic moment in the entire show just happened, out here in the lobby.

Back to the Show

Where were we? Oh yes, in the middle of the fifth act, the one where the patient gets so sick that even their doctor knows for sure. You might think that the action is over, but we're not really done yet, at least not in Maharishi Vedic Science, because it is here that diagnosis gets really fascinating, because there might not be only one clear cause of your illness. It may be that with all that fence-jumping by thug doshas the patient has all kinds of cross influences rumbling around in there and their illness is a bit of a mutt.

We've had the luxury of following the illnesses of Tard and Sikntard from the beginning, but what if they don't make it to the doctor before they are "sick?" What if they wait until it's obvious to get help? In other words, what if the patient is like 99% of the people in the world: they wait until things go bad and then the physician has to take a guess at all of the history back to that overdose of peanut butter and chocolate in Act One.

It takes a skillful diagnostician to sort out all of the plot lines at this point, since the complexity of the story may be increased by combinations of imbalances from different doshas, varying degrees of dhatu, mala, and bad boy srota problems here and there, and all kinds of ama floating around, all of which can result in apparently contradictory symptoms.

Plus with all of those different kinds of tissue in the body, (rasa, rakta, mamsa, medha, ashtii, majja and shukra) your disease could have come from anywhere and be going everywhere else.

Let's just say that this is an exciting stage in the drama, even for the doctor trained in Maharishi Vedic Medicine, and very important, because it would be better for Tard and Sikntard to cut this show short right now by getting well.

Act Six:

This act is called Bheda or "difference." What this means that our patients are so sick they are clearly different from other people. Very sick for one thing.

If the drama of their illness has six acts, it has gone on too long. More than one act is really too long, but we're working on it. But if they don't get things patched up in Act Five, they can only hope for some prolongation of life, but without a return to good health, or they may be differentiated entirely from others, in other words, the bad guys win and they might have to say good-bye to that body they've been living in.

But we suggest that they cut the drama of their illness short long before it shortens their life. And we do that with the effective diagnosis and treatment methods of Maharishi Vedic Medicine.
The following chart summarizes the drama that these two have gone through in becoming ill. One more look at this and then on to the good news.

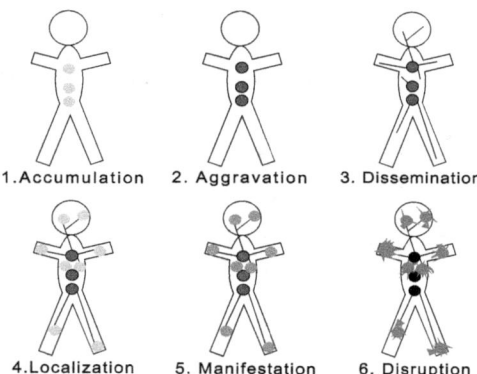

1.Accumulation   2. Aggravation   3. Dissemination

4.Localization   5. Manifestation   6. Disruption

CHAPTER 6

Personal Diagnosis, Customized Cure

Diagnosis : Getting Personal

That drama was informative in a general way about illness in general, but what about chronic fatigue? And since doctors trained in Maharishi Vedic Medicine have certainly diagnosed and treated people with chronic fatigue, what abnormalities do they see in diagnosing such people? What are they looking for? What kinds of questions will they ask?

Usually such diagnosis comes down to noting ama in the system, but you can get that way in many ways. Also, ama in the system may be secondary to other disorders, so it is important to treat those, too.

From the perspective of Maharishi Vedic Medicine, chronic fatigue is generally a vata disorder, a kapha disorder, or a vata-kapha disorder. The general causes are weak digestion, ama, overweight, chronic stress, depression, any disease that has not been attended to, anemia, and old age.

We'll be looking at dietary and behavioral means of addressing these problems, en masse, in upcoming chapters. But the Maharishi Vedic Medicine physician must determine how these imbalances got started.

Too much kapha can create ama. Too much vata can overload the system, creating discoordination in the flow of intelligence through the body, resulting in poor levels of energy. Too much pitta can result in "burning" of the dhatus, the tissues that build the other tissues, which means that you get poorly formed tissues, with ama as a by-product.

You can have dhatuksheya, or diminution of the dhatus, or ojaksheya, lessening of ojas. Ojas is said to be one of the first things that is affected by stress. You can be affected by a diet that decreases the quality of the tissues, slowly leaching health out of the system. Maybe you have been eating foods that are too heavy for your digestive fire to process, such as meat, leftovers, stale or cold food, junk food and peanut butter. That results in more ama.

Whatever the cause, and whatever the condition you are in, just looking at your illness is not likely to give the full picture, which means that just treating your symptoms suffers from the same superficiality. In a way, medicine like that is like building safety nets at the bottom of a ravine to catch people who have fallen off a cliff. We can keep improving the nets, altering the strength, tension, location, etc. The idea of Maharishi Vedic Medicine is to keep people from falling off the cliff in the first place.

To get a picture of just how you fell, got pushed, or jumped into the abyss, the Maharishi Vedic Physician (MVP) will look at a number of factors in evaluating your condition (and how you got there) in order to create a treatment plan to bring you back to vitality.

First of all, you'll probably fill out some forms and then answer a few questions in the presence of a nurse or physician trained in Maharishi Vedic Medicine. Your age must be considered, since age is typically a factor in determining your physical strength and physiological functioning. Different ages are considered to be predominantly kapha (youth), pitta (adolescence/adulthood), and vata (maturity/old age). Doshic aspects of age may contribute to a determination of how you became fatigued.

Your weight is a factor, since overweight is an obvious indicator of metabolic or food intake problems, and underweight/emaciation can be the cause of many diseases.

Your date and place of birth are important considerations to the physician, because the influence of the "Cosmic Counterparts" (see chapter on Jyotish Astrology, below) on your basic constitution and on the current situation that you are experiencing may be of crucial importance in understanding your physiological makeup, what you are going through, and various performances ("yagyas" - see below) that may improve your situation.

The history of any diseases that you may have previously experienced, plus your current symptoms are important factors, not only to find out what's bothering you, but to further establish the nature and functioning of your particular body type, and perhaps establish the factors that may have led to your current state of imbalanced and vitiated doshas and dhatus.

Your personal habits, such as smoking and consumption of alcohol, are factors that will aid the physician in determining the degree to which behavioral factors are weakening your system.

Family histories of genetic disorders or predisposition to depression, overweight, or other factors can be useful indicators of your physiological predisposition.

Your dietary habits, especially habits that would be considered ama-producing (as described above), are also important elements to consider in structuring an accurate diagnosis and successful cure.

Your digestive capacity, e.g. - how long after meals you feel hungry again, whether you feel heavy, tired, or have gas after meals... all this will give clear diagnostic information to the MVP in determining how your bodily machinery is performing the digestive function - which is a crucial factor in your overall health-producing machinery.

The build of your body is indicative of primary constitution. Obviously if you are overweight, you are likely to either have a kapha constitution or at least a kapha imbalance. If you are not a kapha type but still have tremendous fatigue and lethargy, the physician will have to look elsewhere.

Many diseases are related to bowel movement irregularities, so you will probably get questions about that. If you are depressed, moving slowly, and are low on energy, there is a good chance that your elimination is no record-setting process, either. Urination patterns will be a concern as well, in terms of the frequency, color, flow, any burning or incontinence, etc.

The number of hours that you sleep, the time of sleep, interruptions in sleep, regularity, position during sleep (e.g. - sleeping on the stomach, together with grinding of the teeth and an itchy anus could be an indicator of parasites) are all important factors.

Poor routine is an obvious factor, and a contributor to a host of diseases. Some diseases occur more often during certain seasons.

Where you live may be a factor for obvious reasons: ventilation, light, potential environmental toxins, cleanliness and orderliness. And it may a factor for reasons that Maharishi Mahesh Yogi has brought back to light under the auspices of Maharishi Sthapatyaved, the science of proper architectural orientation, proportions and the internal construction of buildings such that they support maximum evolution and health for the inhabitants (see chapter 13).

If you are a woman, the regularity, flow (duration, quantity), associated symptoms (pain, fluid retention, headache, depression, etc.) of your menstrual period is a consideration, as well as any discharge between menstruations, or discontinued menses due to menopause or other reasons.

All of these factors must be considered, among others. For the chronically fatigued patient it may also be necessary to run many of those traditional diagnostic tests that were described in the first chapter. Even so, the answers to these questions will provide enough information for trained practitioners to make an initial assessment of your body type.

At this point, a Maharishi Vedic Physician will perform a procedure of Nadi Vigyan or pulse diagnosis. Pulse diagnosis, when performed by a trained MVP diagnostician, can determine the predominance and vitality of the vata, pitta, or kapha elements in the body, plus give an instant blueprint or snapshot of your current state of health or non-health. It is a surprisingly effective tool, in the right hands.

It might seem odd that one's pulse could contain detailed diagnostic information, but consider the following:

"The body... if it is a pattern of intelligence rather than a heap of material, might be expected to contain enormous amounts of information about the whole in all or at least many of its parts (this is of course true of DNA, for example)."[18]

We have discussed that from the perspective of physics the entire creation is just a manifestation of apparent fluctuations in quantum wave functions, emergent from a single unified field. It makes sense, therefore, to view our physical bodies as combinations of such vibratory wave functions. So, the pulse could be seen to potentially give information about the basic vibrational qualities that make up the physiology, which we have been referring to as vata, pitta, and kapha.

Just as measuring neurological activity informs us of how we're functioning, pulse diagnosis, in competent hands, gives a snapshot of the doshic balance or imbalance that you are living with. This can often reveal the likely origin of your fatigue and guide the diagnostician in selecting behavioral and dietary adjustments that

---

18. H. Sharma and C. Clark, Contemporary Ayurveda
(New York: Churchill Livingstone, 1998), p. 55

you should begin immediately, plus a number of specific treatments uniquely suited to help lift you out of your fatigued condition.

The delight of this type of diagnosis is that it is completely customized for you. It could be said that from the perspective of Maharishi Vedic Medicine, there is no such thing as fatigue. There is only your fatigue. There is no Chronic Fatigue Syndrome. There is only your particular experience and manifestation of Chronic Fatigue Syndrome.

In other words, despite the existence of identifiable conditions and illnesses in general, it is the manifestation of such an illness in your particular physiology that creates a fascinating interplay of your particular strengths, weaknesses, doshic constitution and imbalances with the emerging expression of an "illness." Unravelling that story is the job of the MVM diagnostician. And the good news is that such deep analysis lays the groundwork for deeper cure.

Of course, Rome wasn't built in a day. You probably got your fatigue due to conditions that were in operation over a long period of time, even if the onset of symptoms was sudden. There are modalities of Maharishi Ayurveda that offer instant relief for various ailments (see chapter 15, on Maharishi Vedic Vibration Therapy), but at the same time, you may need to be patient with the re-enlivenment of your physiology. If you have been beating your body into submission with dietary and behavioral imbalances for years, it may take some time to bring it back to full bloom. It will come back, in all likelihood, but it won't happen without cooperation, and some patience, from your side.

In some ways it's much easier to take a pill than it is to go to bed on time. Changing habits is a lot more challenging than miracle cures. Usually changing habits is a lot cheaper, of course, but you will need to take some responsibility for digging out of that hole you dug yourself into.

At the same time Maharishi Vedic Medicine is ready, willing, and able to strengthen you from within, educate you on the climb, and give you a boost up to the light of day. With a little personal diagnostic help from a trained Maharishi Vedic Physician, and a few interesting treatment methods. That's next on our list.

Cure: They're Singing Your Tune

If you are one of those people who likes to get to the bottom line, perhaps you opened to this section first. This is where the good news starts, where we turn from examining how you dug yourself into a hole and start talking about the way back up to the light.

But it's not just about good news. This book is not intended to soothe you with abstractions or positive thinking. Chronic Fatigue is serious stuff. In our experience, people with chronic fatigue have often been suffering for months or even years, and can't deal with their life, their jobs, families, etc. Yet once they start the treatments of Maharishi Vedic Medicine, they quickly become normal people.

We want to emphasize that any degree of chronic fatigue can be helped by this approach. Specifically, with Maharishi Vedic Medicine, chronic fatigue can be cured, and Chronic Fatigue Syndrome can be helped, and possibly cured.

In our experience, this treatment offers a unique opportunity for chronically fatigued patients to feel better in a matter of weeks or months. Chronic Fatigue Syndrome is certainly a more serious condition, and we suggest that if you have CFS you will need supervised Maharishi Vedic Medicine treatment on an in or out-patient basis.

But Maharishi Vedic Medicine will help in either case, because it is not a symptom-based treatment. Your symptoms will be treated, too, since the underlying causes will be treated. But using band-aid treatments on individual symptoms just delays the process of healing and recovery.

The underlying strength or bala of your physiology must be shored up first, which is the approach of Maharishi Vedic Medicine.

For both chronic fatigue and Chronic Fatigue Syndrome it's best to see a doctor. The treatments that we will be describing in the remainder of this book are examples of what may be prescribed for chronic fatigue (i.e. simple changes in diet, exercise, daily routine, etc.). CFS, on the other hand, is a complex, multi-system disease that requires a multi-dimensional approach.

Make no mistake, however, the treatments described here will aid in lessening symptoms and even support the cure or remission of CFS. But CFS typically requires a more long term treatment, since the doctor must both address and redress the level of agni(s), the digestion, the bowel movements, and complicating factors such as arthritis, fevers, etc.

Memory

In general, all of the curative elements that we will soon be discussing are about what we could call memory, which is termed "smriti" in Maharishi Vedic Medicine. Memory in this context means remembering who you really are. We established that you are really an entity brimming with consciousness, made, in effect, out of a transcendental field of unlimited energy and intelligence.

Since that is the case, bringing you back to health is simply bringing you back home to where you really belong, your source, your origin, your true nature. Since that is the case, a cure of this nature is just that, completely natural. But it's not automatic. You've unintentionally worked and overworked very hard over a long period of time to get yourself in the situation you are in, and it takes a while to bring you back home, to remind yourself of who you really are, and to reacquaint yourself with your birthright, which is to live life in perfect health, perfect happiness and fulfillment.

The remaining chapters in this book will discuss various forms of memory booster, i.e. ways that your mind and body can be reminded of their essential nature and reset to that pristine, powerful, healthy state. Just as we can reset a computer to start over when some program has misfired or crashed, we now can begin to reset your physiology to do what it was originally supposed to do. We'll be cleaning out your system, getting rid of bugs, improving resistance to viruses, and reprogramming your physiological computer with the original software.

To do that we will have to reopen the flow of intelligence to the parts of the body that have been lacking proper connections. For some reason, nourishment/intelligence/energy has not been reaching your entire body and you feel fatigued. Maybe there has been a lack of integration between body and mind, improper nourishment, an imbalance of agni, too much ama, or not enough ojas.

You may be undernourished, malnourished, or overfed. You may have blocked srotas, and lack strength, feel dull, have body aches, flatulency, regurgitations, indigestion, food just sitting there in your digestive system. Anything could be happening.

Whatever the condition, we usually will be dealing with elevated ama in the system, along with, most likely, some derangement of agni, the digestive fire. We need to reduce ama and normalize the functions of agni.

We need to establish a greater connection between you and the inner intelligence of your own physiology. Your body is constantly sending out signals of what it likes and doesn't like, but have you been listening? If you are cut off from your body's inner intelligence, it's probably because you never knew it existed, or you ignored the messages, not realizing their importance.

Those days are over. Your body is dying to tell you what's good for it. As a matter of fact, if it can't get your attention, it may get sick and tired of trying. But that, at least, you can feel. Sick and tired you can understand. But this is no way to get along with what should be your best friend. Why wait until your friend is dead tired and chronically sick to tell them that you care?

We're going to repair that relationship with special treatments to clean out those srotas. We're going to clean out and nourish the digestive tract. We're going to use oil massage to start the flow of intelligence throughout the body. We'll learn some new easy, exercises that will get your body moving together again. We'll ask your help in modifying your behavior, diet, daily and seasonal schedules, and even see if you can dredge up some will power to start behaving in ways that will put your life back in tune with the natural laws of the universe the only set of laws that make you feel good when you live by them, not just punishing you when you blow it.

We're going to suggest techniques that will bring you back to health from the angle of the mind, body and behavior. Your active cooperation and proper exercise of your will, of choice, choosing to do what you know is good for you, will make all this easier.

All in all, however, you are simply being asked to remember who you are, and the treatments, dutifully followed, will only be bringing you closer to home, closer to your true nature.

It's the strangest thing to think that there is a medicine which knows you better than you do, but that is exactly what Maharishi Vedic Medicine is about. I'm not saying that a Maharishi Vedic Medicine knows the ins and outs of your experiences, what you did today, how you stubbed your toe when you were six, etc. That's not it.

Rather, imagine that you are walking into a store filled with medicated oils, bottled nutritive pills of various kinds, spices, soaps, shampoos, aroma bottles, candles, and other supplies. In this store there are vata pacifying spices, oils that are soothing to the dryer skin of men over 40, special teas to pacify Kapha, herbs to soothe that effects of menopause, and special "rasayanas" or elixirs that are powerful anti-oxidants to counteract aging.

What's different about such a store in comparison to any health store? This store carries herbs that are designed to remind you of who you are. These stores exist in the real world, of course, under the name Health and Wholeness, and they feature Maharishi Ayurveda Products. But the fascinating thought that I have when I walk into these stores is that is that their products are unlike anything you can find anywhere else in the world, since, at least on a conceptual level, some of these products are as if whispering to me. Whispering my true nature.

That may seem a bit poetic, and it is, but it's also scientific, since these herbal products are said to have an actual vibrational quality, which is chosen for its medicinal effect. I'll talk more about this later in my chapter on herbs, but the principle is that an herb is a wave function of the infinite field, just like you are.

These herbs have identifiable qualities of vata, pitta and kapha, just like you do. And some herbs, as vibrating aspects of cosmic intelligence, are vibrating at a frequency and a note which, in some cases, are the notes at which you should be vibrating. The herbs haven't forgotten what you have forgotten. The herbs didn't stay up late partying and drinking, or working until the wee hours, or eating what's wrong, or worrying over nothing much. The herbs are still ringing the notes that you should be ringing. You can't really hear the song they are singing to you when you walk in the door. But you should know it's there.

And by using the right herbs and oils, by beginning the proper diet, changing to a healthier routine, (as recommended by your Maharishi Ayurveda expert) and by experiencing your true, unbounded nature through the Transcendental Meditation Program, you are resetting your physiology to its true, primordial attunement with the cosmic symphony, and perfect health cannot help but be supported on that basis.

More on this note in the following chapters.

CHAPTER 7

The Transcendental Meditation Program[tm]: A Gentle Reminder

If you don't know what "TM" is, the first question is, where have you been? If you haven't heard of the Transcendental Meditation Program[tm], brought to the west by Maharishi Mahesh Yogi in the 1960's, you must have been very busy, working overtime at the office.

Yes, by now, many books have been written on the topic, over 400 research studies have been published all over the world, and the effects of this simple yet profound technique have been well-documented in the areas of stress reduction, blood pressure normalization, increased intelligence, improved relations with co-workers and supervisors, quicker reaction time, self-actualization, and even some sociological factors such as effects of group meditation on crime rate and reduction of violence in war zones.[19]

It's all there, highly documented and scientifically supported. The Transcendental Meditation Program[tm] is possibly the most thoroughly examined and documented physiological/psychological phenomenon in modern scientific literature.

But the question is, what's in it for you?

First of all, you might like some of the studies that I didn't mention, like increased energy, deep state of relaxation, reduction of

19. Orme-Johnson, Alexander, et al., Journal of Conflict Resolution, 32(4), 776-812, 1988; Orme-Johnson, Alexander, & Davies, Journal of Conflict Resolution, 34(4), 756-768, 1990

insomnia, reduced dependence on alcohol and cigarettes, decreased use of non-prescription drugs, lessened anxiety, etc. Those sound like something that chronically fatigued people would enjoy.

But the main thing that I'd like to mention, first off, is deep rest. That's right, TM brings profound state of deep rest to the physiology.

That I would bring this up is of course no news to Maharishi Mahesh Yogi, who first brought the TM program to the West in 1958. At that time he was following up on an impulse to bring the blessings of the knowledge of his own spiritual teacher, (long title coming up here) His Divinity Swami Brahmananda Saraswati, Shankarcharya of Jyotir-Math, to the non-monks of the world.

And what was that knowledge? The knowledge of how to easily and effortlessly contact the inner reservoir of pure energy and intelligence and deeply infuse that field of pure consciousness into the mind and body so as to automatically maintain and experience that enlightened state in the midst of practical, everyday life, forever established in and enjoying higher states of consciousness.

But in L.A. it was announced by the press as a wonderful sleep aid.

Even though such a categorization severely under-represents the potential benefits of the Transcendental Meditation Program™, even very, very tired people are welcome and able to experience the benefits.

In English, we have a number of ways of expressing this. You have to start somewhere. Rome wasn't built in a day. A journey of a thousand miles starts with one step.

However we say it, the point is that the technique of TM brings a profound state of rest to the physiology, and the effects are cumulative over time. Now, the last time I checked, we were talking in this book about an ailment where people hardly ever feel rested, where they can't get a good night's sleep, where they wake up feeling almost as exhausted as when they went to bed.

By adding another cycle of rest to your day, which is in addition deeply calming to the mind and rejuvenating to your physiology, you are doing wonderful things to counteract chronic fatigue, which, after all, might be expected to respond positively to a new, dynamic form of rest that addresses both physical fatigue and mental stress.

It may be that long standing, deeper stresses and strains are keeping you from feeling rested after a night's sleep. Maybe the old technique of just sleeping it off isn't enough to handle the complex stressful inputs that our nervous systems are subject to in modern life. Maybe we need a more dynamic state of rest to handle the more dynamic situations that modern living throws at us.

That's the Transcendental Meditation Program™.
After all, what does the Transcendental Meditation Program™ do but bring you back home to what you really are? It is a simple, natural technique that allows the conscious mind to experience finer and finer aspects of a thought, and having transcended that, arrive at the source of thought.

Source of thought? That's a whole discussion of its own.

How Does It Work?

To understand the source of thought concept and how that makes the Transcendental Meditation Program™ possible, we have to talk about thought itself, which is something that we don't usually discuss, or even think about.

A thought can be seen to have energy, of a sort, since it seems to move somewhere. Its a kind of impulse. Thoughts exhibit intelligence, since they move in a particular direction. A thought, therefore, is an impulse of energy and intelligence.

Having established that (stay with me here), we might ask, where do thoughts come from? Most people would agree that they seem to emerge from deep within the mind. And, of course, most of us have many, many thoughts in a day, certainly in the thousands.

Having established that thoughts are an impulse of energy and intelligence, and that we have thousands of them popping up in the mind every day, you might surmise that there must be some source of these thoughts. And if there is a source of thought, deep in the mind, you might think that that source would be a great, perhaps unlimited source of energy and intelligence.

Of course, from the perspective of Maharishi Vedic Medicine, what we are calling the source of thought, the unlimited reservoir of energy and intelligence, is nothing other that the pure field of consciousness that we described earlier as underlying all of life.

In other words, deep inside your own mind, you have access, through the Transcendental Meditation Program™, to your own true essential nature, free of pragyaparadh (mistake of the intellect), free of all limitation, suffering and fatigue.

It's a great field of life, it's your own true source and essential nature, and now you can take a 20 minute vacation to visit it, twice a day, through the Transcendental Meditation Program™.

We need to make one more point to show you how natural all this is. No additives. No side effects. The point is that this whole process, the technique of the Transcendental Meditation Program™, happens due to the mind's natural tendency to want to enjoy more.

To see this point, let's consider, first of all, what drives your mind from topic to topic? Is the mind like a monkey, jumping from one thing to the next, never satisfied? Yes, in some ways that's true. But what drives the monkey from branch to branch, tree to tree?

The pursuit of happiness. The mind is effortlessly drawn to what charms it. If you are reading a quantum physics book and your favorite tune comes on the radio, it takes no effort for the mind to switch from the physics to the lovely tune. And then when the mind remembers that potential delight of a good grade in physics, it will easily find its way back to the book.

This natural tendency of the mind to move in the direction of greater happiness allows the Transcendental Meditation Program™ to work, since the technique allows the conscious mind of the individual to remain active, yet not busy on the level of meaning. The individual is given a sound, called a "mantra," which is a Sanskrit word, the meaning of which is unimportant, and by applying the proper technique of using it, the mind is naturally drawn to the source of thought within.

This is due to the fact that the source of thought, as an infinite reservoir of energy and intelligence, is naturally charming to the mind, and so it is drawn there with no effort, once the busy activity of the mind is disengaged.

It's this use of the natural tendency of the mind that makes the Transcendental Meditation Program™ so natural, completely effortless, and suitable for practical people. It doesn't require powerful capabilities of concentration. It doesn't involve concentration or even contemplation at all. You don't have to be an intellectual, or sit in any unusual positions. Its just a simple, natural process.

But its simplicity doesn't mean that its not powerful. Sometimes the simplest things are the most profound. And this is the granddaddy of that "sometimes."

So, what's in it for you? I think that we could make quite a list here.

First of all, we talked earlier in this book about how you got sick in the first place, how, on some primordial level, all sickness is due to disconnection from the field of pure consciousness, which is your true self. Well, what if you could pay a visit to your true nature, twice a day?

It's been 20, 30, 40 years or more that you've been moving around, with no clear connection to your true nature. Don't you think a visit to your true self would do you good?

If you experience, even for a short while, your true nature, which is pure consciousness, maybe you would start to remember who you really are a bit more. Remember how we said that the reality of "cure" is simply memory of your true nature, and that all of the modalities of Maharishi Vedic Medicine are there simply to remind you of your essential nature and to disassociate your identification with the mirage of illness which has taken over your experience?

Is it any wonder why there is still such an emphasis on the Transcendental Meditation Program™, in Maharishi Vedic Medicine? Sure, we have expert diagnosis from certified MD's, we have herbs and oil massage treatments, advice on diet, behavior, daily routine, and even recommendations on where to live.

But is it any surprise that a technique which takes you straight to an undifferentiated field of pure consciousness, which is also considered to have the attributes of pure happiness, unbounded bliss consciousness, unlimited energy and intelligence, infinite creativity, among other fine qualities, would be highly recommended for a tired person like you?

It's obvious. That's why this chapter is called "A Gentle Reminder."

We all need reminding of our true inner nature. When you think about it, it's easy to go wrong, because we are as if born in the middle of a bunch of insistent distractions as part of the human package.

These distractions are known as sight, touch, taste, hearing, and smell. That's right, our senses have been clamoring for our attention since day one. The sense organs are our means of experience, typically. So our attention is naturally drawn out into the world of experience.

We don't come with an "inner" ear, which naturally draws us to the inner field of pure consciousness. We live in consciousness, but nowadays we have to be reminded how to find it in its true nature. There's a great pair of lines in a poem, "Sailing to Byzantium," by William Butler Yeats that say:

"Caught in that sensual music all neglect Monuments of unageing intellect"

And that, extending the metaphor, is us, typically, lost in the sensual music of experience, without access to our inner nature.

Gaining access to that, innocently, easily, through the Transcendental Meditation Program™, begins to set the physiology right and in the direction to holistic growth back to perfect health.

It's as if you can visit perfect health, twice a day, at least with your mind. However, since the mind and body are intimately connected, when the mind settles down, the body settles down, too. So, while the mind is experiencing deep calm, the body experiences a deep state of relaxation.

This resetting of the mind and body to a more optimal style of functioning, even if only twice a day, even in the midst of the life of a chronically fatigued patient, has the effect of strengthening the patient, bringing at least some rest to the situation. Most importantly, it creates a basis for the other treatment modalities to work.

We can pull a table across the room while holding on any leg. We can improve your fatigued state by working on the level of the mind, body, behavior and environment. In Maharishi Vedic Medicine, we work on all of these levels at the same time, but we suggest that you start building from the ground state up, giving yourself a head start in your quest for energy and health by experiencing the pure field of infinite energy and intelligence, which is nothing other your own true nature, through the Transcendental Meditation Program^{tm}.

There are advanced techniques of the Transcendental Meditation Program^{tm}, and related practices such as the TM-Sidhis Program^{tm}, and even a number of studies that indicate improvement in society through the group practice of the TM and TM-Sidhis programs, used in combination. But we're going to start with the basics, clearing up your fatigue, and work up to the more expansive possibilities over time.

And to build a foundation for such exalted development, we're going to start with the mundane, i.e. - we're going to have to restructure your day.

CHAPTER 8

Ideal Routine, or Simple Healing Requiring Only Diligence, Fortitude, Rescheduling, and Some Dietary Changes

Let's face it, you need to see a doctor. If you are chronically fatigued, I think that you can see from what we've talked about thus far that there are many potential reasons why you have arrived in this reduced state of health. You need to get a customized roadmap out of the wastelands that you have driven into. If you are in the grips of CFS, you don't need me to tell you that need medical attention. Your body is letting you know every day.

Even so, even though you would be wise to consult with a trained Maharishi Vedic Medicine physician, there are things you can do to start the ball rolling in a healthy direction, simply on the level of what you do every day. These behavioral changes can directly contribute to the strengthening and rejuvenation of your physiology and get you started back up the road to health.

One advantage about reading about these things here, before you may have spoken to an MVM physician, is that you will already be familiar with many aspects of the physician's "prescription" for you. Much of what I will talk about in this chapter will be present or at least touched on in the instructions you receive from the doctor.

I'll bet that you could write a good portion of that prescription and this chapter yourself. Much of what I have to tell you is common sense, or at least folk wisdom, such as "early to bed, early to rise," and other such sayings. I don't have to tell you that staying up late is killing you. I don't need to tell you that a harried, complex, constantly changing schedule of work, food and sleep is draining you.

But maybe you would like to know why. I don't know about you, but when I had an authority figure answer my questions regarding moral imperatives with "because I say so," it never had as much weight as when I understood the principle behind the precept.

So here are some principles.

First of all, you may have heard of the term circadian rhythms. Circadian means, literally, "around the day." They are the rhythms of the nervous system and the physiology that we progress through each day as we move from waking up, through work, hunger, more work, exhaustion, and back to sleep.

Maharishi Vedic Medicine is all over this topic, with a discipline called dinacharya ("din" being related to our word "day" and "acharya" meaning teacher or knowledge). Dinacharya means the knowledge of daily schedule. An expanded version of this study is called Ritucharya, the knowledge of Ritu, or seasonal schedules.

Dinacharya doesn't fall far from the tree that we've been climbing all of this time, since Maharishi Vedic Medicine identifies certain times of day that correspond to vata, pitta and kapha doshas. The vata time of day is said to be from 2:00 to 6:00, the kapha time of day is 6:00 to 10:00, while pitta rules 10:00 to 2:00. When you consider that these cover both a.m. and p.m., they've got it covered all day.

Let's look at the implications of this typology for understanding the importance of daily routine in restructuring your health.

Okay, it's two in the morning, and vata starts up. Hopefully you are sleeping at this time. If not, you will probably start to wake up even more than you wanted, and find it difficult to get to sleep. If, however, you went to bed in good time, there is a good chance that you will wake up sometime between two and six a.m., since, in that time frame, all of nature is waking up, the birds are chirping away, the air is fresh, and if you have a window open, or if you have ever gone camping, that fresh air is going to sneak into your dreams like an alarm clock and pop you right awake.

And it's a good thing, too, because if you sleep through into the six a.m. or beyond, it is kapha time, all of a sudden you are going to crash again. If you get up before six, you are waking up with nature, and the mind and body receive a wave of fresh energy to start the day.

That phrase "a wave of fresh energy" should ring some alarm bells for the chronically fatigued. Your mind should be saying this: "Fresh energy. Good."

But if you sleep past 6 a.m., you will find that more of the kapha qualities of dullness and lethargy creep into your mind and physiology. I think you may have plenty of that already. No need to stock up.

On the other hand, if you are up, the time from 6 to 10 a.m. (and p.m.) is a great time for exercise. Of course, if you are a CFS patient, you better start slowly. You are already slow, so that's no problem. Just don't make any sudden moves, since exercise for most CFS people is extremely challenging. So you might start with a walk of about fifty steps. Then you might be able to do one set of an exercise called Suryanamaskar, or Sun Salutation (described below, or even easier).

I'm going to talk about exercise in detail later, but at least you now know the best time to do it.

From 10 to noon and on to 2 p.m. should be your sharpest time of day. Pitta rules mental clarity, sharpness, and of course, digestive fire. This is the time when digestive capability is at its peak, and it is, therefore, the time when you should eat your main meal of the day.

For many people, this appears to require a major lifestyle change. You are on the go all day, lunch is a bagel and coffee, and you really eat at night. That may have been your situation, but, to put it indelicately, those days are over! You said you wanted to feel good again, didn't you? You, of all people, who probably have an ama condition in your physiology, you whose digestive mechanism is obviously not doing very well at its core job of producing ojas (which is experienced as happiness, vitality, etc.), you need as much help digesting food as possible.

It's time to get creative here. If you want to eat your big meal in the middle of the day, you will find a way. You'll do some of the prep work the night before. You'll bring more in your lunch bucket. You'll make it so.

By the way, it's also important that you eat in a settled atmosphere. You shouldn't feel rushed. Think of your digestion as a sort of bonfire. You wouldn't want to put it in a windy place. You would do best to protect it in a stable fireplace, or at least put some big rocks around it. You wouldn't get an efficient fire if every few minutes you pushed it around with a shovel from here to there.

It's also important that you give your attention to what you are eating, and that you either maintain silence or engage in uplifting conversation while you eat. It's widely known that negative thinking reduces your energy and vitality. You don't want be adding negativity to the equation when you are having food, which, in way, is a form of new energy coming into your life.

The other reason for calm in the dining room is so that you can listen. It might seem odd to talk of listening while eating, but we have established that your physiology is brimming with intelligence, and we also have discussed that if you are in tune with your own inner intelligence, you will probably choose behaviors and foods that are likely to be better for your particular physiology.

So, while you are eating, your body may actually be "speaking" to you, in a way, telling you what is best for you to eat, and how much of each. If we are not listening to our own inner intelligence, there is no way that we can expect to grow healthier. So listen up, and eat right.
One extra tip about diet is that you should not eat to your maximum capacity. That is considered to overload the physiology such that your pitta cannot handle it all, and digestion will be partial and more

ama will result. Maharishi Vedic Medicine recommends that you eat to 3/4 of your capacity, which can be estimated as the amount of food that you could hold in your two hands cupped together.

After lunch you go into that vata period again, two to six p.m., a good time for mental work, but sometimes a bit of a slump. Late afternoon, therefore, is a great time to do your second Transcendental Meditation Program of the day. Then, going into the evening, you will have released the stresses of the day, and you can use the evening (kapha) time to wind down so that you get to bed before ten.

This is that "early to bed, early to rise" thing coming back to visit you. As it turns out, Mother was right, but we said that we'd tell you why. And the "why" is that if you don't get to bed before ten, you will almost certainly find yourself getting what appears to be a second wind, mentally. Suddenly the slowness of the evening is replaced by a burning need to finish off those bills, by a letter you just have to write, by that sonnet you haven't finished (poets only), and you will stay up until midnight or beyond, either catching up on the day or apparently getting ahead of the next.

Unfortunately, the energy that you are running on is intended to fuel another project entirely, which is the physiological cleanup crew. That's right, according to Maharishi Vedic Medicine, the hours from 10 p.m. until 2 a.m. are supposed to be utilized by the body to burn off impurities that have gathered in the physiology all day, and to clean out the kapha in body and mind so that you can start the next day afresh

But if you are working the body and mind in that time period, the clean up crew never gets a chance to do its best work. Then junk starts to build up in the corners, a little trash here, a little gunk there, and pretty soon your body doesn't function as smoothly as it used to, the corridors (srotas, remember) are clogged, and you start to feel fatigued all of the time.

You can see how things get all mixed up. You feel more alert at night. You are fatigued all day. Something is wrong here. Any accomplishment seems like a good thing. But tonight's accomplishment at the expense of tomorrow's happiness is just robbing Peter and then not being able to pay Paul. Something got lost there.

This brings up the major problem with the typical "big meal at night" thing, which is that pitta is low and kapha is high. What that means, metabolically speaking, is that you are loading up the digestive process with work to do at a time when it is the weakest. Then, at 10 p.m., when the pitta stage sets in, the digestive fire that should be doing its cleanup of the body is redeployed to digesting your dinner.

The result, usually, is that neither function works very well, you neither get your dinner fully digested nor your body deeply rejuvenated. That translates into more ama. Poorly digested food. Unprocessed long-standing impurities hanging around. Is it any wonder your physiological machine is misfiring, losing power, and calling out for an oil change?

So that's what you are going to do. You are going to change your diet.

You are going to change your schedule. You are going to go to bed before ten, even if it means just lying there for a while before falling asleep. You have to start creating some new habits.

It is said to take as much as two weeks for a new habit to stick. So that's all you have to commit to, fourteen days of going to bed before ten, and, at the same time, 14 days of getting up before six. Just keeping to this schedule alone will start you a long way down the road to increased energy.

It works for mental patients. One of the first things that they do for mental patients is to get them on a regular routine. And even though you may not be crazy, your body is, at least, suffering from an extreme, physical form of depression.

That's your daily schedule, at least the basics. Here's a complete list:

Morning
- Arise early in the morning
- Evacuate bowels and bladder
- Clean teeth
- Clean or scrape tongue
- Oil massage to head, body, and soles of feet (details below)
- Cut nails if needed
- Gargle with sesame oil
- Bathe or shower
- TM and TM-Sidhi Program
- Exercise according to individual recommendations

- Wear clean and comfortable dress, suitable to season and activity
- Light breakfast (optional), depending upon constitutional type
- Work or study

Afternoon

- Lunch: Diet balanced according to constitutional type and individual Recommendations
- Brief rest after lunch
- Work or study
- Transcendental Meditation Program and TM-Sidhi Program

Evening

- Light supper: Diet balanced according to constitutional type and individual recommendations
- Pleasant, relaxing activity (e.g. an evening walk)
- Early to bed

One item on that list deserves a special mention, and that is scraping the tongue, first thing in the morning. If you want to see ama up close and personal, you can observe it in the form of the white coating on your tongue in the morning. When you consider that ama is something that you'd like to get out of your body, I'm sure that you'll see the logic of scraping it off of your tongue rather than recycling it back through the system with your morning toast. Most pharmacies have tongue scrapers. Once you get started on this one it's hard to go back.

I'll be giving details on some more of those items soon, but first I'd like to also discuss the annual or seasonal rhythms of ritucharya.

You might want to know, for example, that spring is basically kapha, wet and cool, while summer is pitta, hot, and winter is vata, cold and dry. So, depending on your particular constitution or dosha type, you may do well to act appropriately in each season.

If you are a kapha type, you may need to exercise more, especially in the spring. If you are pitta, summertime exercise is not your best bet, and vata types had better stay warm in the winter.

Maharishi Vedic Medicine indicates that the physiology actually picks up doshic influences from the season that is underway, and that unless these doshas are cleaned out at the end of the season, the effects of the previous season may carry over into the new season. In other words, summer may be over but your body is somehow still overheated inside way into the fall. This inhibits the flexibility of the metabolism to adjust appropriately to the next season, and may reduce the efficient function of the physiology to the point that these left over doshic effects contribute to the development of ama in the body.

You remember ama. A persistent, yet unwelcome visitor.

It is recommended, therefore, that you take recourse to a regimen of "panchakarma" at the end of each season, so that you can move into the new season afresh. I will be describing this in my next chapter in detail, and once you have experienced it, you will wish that you could do it every month. It is deeply rejuvenating.

One seasonal tip is that you should rest more in winter, going to bed earlier, since winter vitiates vata.

Of course, for most of us, panchakarma comes at the end of one very long season, i.e. our whole life up until now, so there are a lot of doshic imbalances to clear out.

Fortunately the healthy state of the body is more natural, and therefore easier for it to maintain. It's a lot of work for the body to be ill. It's easier for it to be healthy. So, resetting the physiology as healthy is a lot less work than it was to get it sick.

One thing that panchakarma includes that you can start doing at home right away is abhyanga, an oil massage.

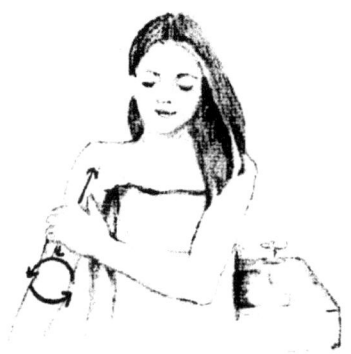

Your panchakarma treatment will feature an in-depth version of this, usually with two highly trained and well-synchronized attendants, but you can do quite a bit of good to yourself, and of course you are there every day, while attendants are more likely to be an occasional thing, for most people.

First of all, there are a wide variety of specialized oils available through Maharishi Ayurvedic Products International,[20] some of them herbalized to suit your particular dosha, or to help with your doshic imbalance. Sesame oil is recommended for vata and kapha constitutions, and coconut oil for pitta. Even olive oil is used, by some people, which can leave you with the fragrance of freshly cooked bread, if you like that sort of thing.

This self-massage is simply performed, usually in the morning, before your shower or bath. If you can heat the oil slightly, it has a more penetrating effect. A small squirt bottle of oil dipped in hot water will quickly heat up a bit.

Some practicalities should be mentioned, in order to integrate this massage into your environment with a minimum of muss and fuss. You should probably sit on a towel to perform the massage, although the massage can also be done standing up. You will want to have some paper towels to wipe excess oil off after you are done. It will probably be best to start some hot water running in the tub or shower to heat up the pipes so that the oil does not stick and cause a blockage. You can leave this water running after the shower as well to help disperse any remaining oil.

Now, an oil massage is a new concept for many of us who established our cleanliness habits in the (pitta) years of our adolescence when a drop of oil on the skin on one day probably meant a blemish the next.

20. www.mapi.com

In the U.S., at least, top to bottom scrubbing is the order of the day. But such scrubbing can strip the natural oils from the skin, and as we mature, we actually need those oils to protect the skin from dryness and undue wrinkling.

So the ayurvedic massage changes some of those scrubbing habits, by suggesting that you cover your body with oil, with a light spreading motion, and then go back over the major portions of head, limbs, chest, torso, legs and feet with a soothing, deep rub. The joints are treated with circular strokes while the flat areas (or what used to be flat) are given long strokes. Special attention is given to the ears, including all of those little inner folds, and to the feet.

If you don't have time to do a complete massage to the head, you can skip it, but the head is one of the best areas to treat, especially for vata disorders. Of course, if you insist on having oil-free hair, there will be a good bit of scrubbing to do, right after the massage.

Washing up after massage includes wiping off excess oil (reduces the load on your drain), and then soaping up mainly your private parts and your under arms, but that is all. The rest of the body should be allowed to keep the benefit of this oil blessing to carry it into the day. Also, if you are having trouble sleeping at night, an abhyanga is a soothing sleep aid.

One bit of practical advice is to be careful if your towels get oily, since they can burst into flame in the dryer if not fully cleansed of oil. You may want to presoak them or even put 1/8 cup of dish detergent in with your regular laundry soap to cut the oil.

Another point is that sesame oil needs to be "cured," or preheated, to make it more penetrating and effective. Curing sesame oil simply means putting it in a pot on medium heat and bringing it up to 212 degrees Fahrenheit, which is the boiling point of water. You can tell if it has hit that level by dropping a few drops of water in the oil, and they will start to crackle when the desired heat is reached. You then cool the oil and it is ready for daily use.

Organic oils are best, and Maharishi Ayur-Ved "Health and Wholeness" stores have an array of such oils, both basic organic sesame oil and herbalized sesame oil formulations suitable for vata, pitta or kapha, rejuvenating oils for women over 40, for men over 40, revitalizing facial oils, a deep muscle rub, and a "joint soothe" oil. (see also MAPI.com).

It's important for CFS patients to remember that although oil massage is good for you, since it reduces vata, stimulates the flow of intelligence through the body, helps develop ojas, cleans toxins out of the body, enlivening the entire physiology, abhyanga at home should be very light and gentle. You should leave the vigorous massage efforts to the Maharishi Vedic Medicine clinicians.

There are other physical things that you can engage in to enliven the inner intelligence of the physiology, such as the suryanamaskar, or "Sun Salutations" and the neuromuscular integration program, which uses a set of physical positions for the body to engage in, commonly called asanas.

The word asana means "seat" since many of these exercises are performed sitting down. For some of you that will sound like "my kind of exercise," but you might want to wait a minute before you start celebrating, because they can get a bit more challenging than it sounds. But not the way we're going to do it.

I'll start by explaining a few of the asanas, and then the suryanamaskar, or sun salute sequence. If you are healthy enough to do the full suryanamaskar ("surya") sequence, that is great, but many CFS patients will find it far from their capabilities, at least at first. For the purposes of the chronically fatigued, I will first describe a few easy asanas can be used as a starting point, and propose an order in which you might want to try them

But first, please note that if you have any kind of back injury or other physical limitation, you need to have a consultation first before engaging in such exercises.

To begin with the easy stuff, even though I said that you may want to wait on the Sun Salutation sequence, you should be able to do the very first part of it, which serves as a beginning to this easy sequence of exercises.

First, stand erect, with your feet close together, and put your palms and fingers together in front of your breastbone. Just gaze forward easily for five seconds. Breathe normally. That's a good start.

But wait, there's more!

Secondly, slowly raise the arms so that they are straight over your head, palms forward, then continue the movement until the arms are slightly behind your head, and you are leaning back a bit from the waist.

From the beginning to the end of this movement you should inhale fully, and hold the breath until you start the next movement. Gaze up at the ceiling or sky, whichever is first. Hold that pose for five seconds.

Thirdly, exhale and lean forward and touch the ground with your palms, hands about shoulder width apart, keeping your knees straight. Okay, now that you're done laughing about being asked to do that, I'll explain.

On this third part just go as far as you can without straining. You'll get more flexible over time. If you can't do this with straight legs, let your knees bend so that you can get your hands on the ground to provide a basis for the next move. Hold that position, or as close as you got, complete with exhaled breath, for five seconds.

Then you can stand up straight again and do a sidebend or chandrasana (crescent moon) pose. To do that you inhale, raise your hands over your head, and while you lean to one side, exhale and press your opposite hip in the other direction. Then repeat for the other side.

You can then sit down on the ground or on an exercise mat on the ground and do a few more things.

First lie on your back and do a "jathara parivartanasana" or spinal twist, which involves putting your arms out to the side in a T shape, then bringing your knees up toward your chest, followed by rotating your torso so that the knees move toward or even rest on the ground at your side. Repeat for the other side

Follow that by straightening out your legs and then resting them on the ground. Then you can bring up one knee at a time and do some light bicycling of your legs in the air, which is called pada sanchalasana or cycling pose.

Then you could move to a do a modified shalabhasana or locust pose. To do this you roll over onto on your stomach and, with your arms at your side, raise one leg and then the other, to whatever degree is comfortable. Advanced practitioners do both legs at one time, but let's not get ahead of the pack just now, unless it's easy.

While you are down there on your stomach, you might also do a cobra or bhujangasana pose, in which you place your hands face down on the floor and begin to lift up your head and torso off the ground, guiding the lift with your hands and arms, but not pushing down with your hands and arms. You may not get off the ground at first but even the intention and some muscular engagement in that direction that is a start.

You could then finish with what is called chetanasana, the world's simplest asana, since you simply lie on your back with feet extended and arms lightly resting at your side, and then put your attention on your whole body. You might do that for 2-3 minutes. This enlivens awareness in the body, and is also relaxing.

Instruction in these specialized exercises will typically be available to you as part of the treatment plan provided in your Maharishi Vedic Medicine prescription.

For those who have more energy, and feel ready to do it, there is the full Suryanamaskar or sun salutation sequence. These "suryas" are integrating and rejuvenating for the whole body, involving the body, mind and breath. Your body is obviously involved, there is a simple breathing pattern that goes along with the physical movement, and just remembering all this will certainly engage the mind! At least until you have done it a few times and then it becomes automatic.

There are 12 positions in one surya, and you hold each position for about 5 seconds. That means that one surya should take about a minute. New CFS patients are recommended to start with the easy sequence of asanas that we described above, or one surya, twice a day, if possible.

That's right, we are asking you to do two minutes of exercise a day. It's a start. Even so, we don't want you to strain, so you should stop and rest if you notice heavy breathing or perspiration, and lie down and rest for a minute or two.

This rest period advice doesn't apply if you break out into a sweat at the very thought of exercise. If it makes you feel better you could ahead and think of resting for a few seconds, but, after all, that kind of routine is all in your mind. So, let's get back to the suryas.

By the way, if you can face the sun while you do this you would be doing an actual sun "salute." It wouldn't hurt if you could actually see the sun, or even better, if you could be out in the fresh air and sunlight. On the other hand, it might make the neighbors gawk, and of course, direct sunlight might be hard to come by in your section of the condo. In any case, don't look directly at the sun while you do this, for obvious reasons, you are getting a free dose of vitamin D.

How to do suryanamaskar, a new kind of 12 step program:

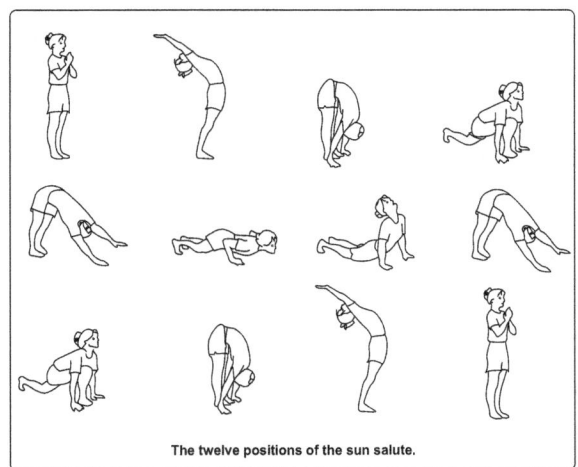

The twelve positions of the sun salute.

First, as we said earlier, stand erect, with your feet close together, and put your palms and fingers together in front of your breastbone. Just gaze forward easily for five seconds. Breathe normally.

Secondly, slowly raise the arms so that they are straight over your head, palms forward, then continue the movement until the arms are slightly behind your head, and you are leaning back a bit from the waist.

From the beginning to the end of this movement you should inhale fully, and hold the breath until you start the next movement. Gaze up at the ceiling/sky. Hold that pose for five seconds.

Thirdly, exhale and lean forward and touch the ground with your palms, hands about shoulder width apart, keeping your knees straight.

Just go as far as you can without straining. If you can't do this with straight legs, let your knees bend so that you can get your hands on the ground to provide a basis for the next move. Hold that position, or as close as you got, complete with exhaled breath, for five seconds

Fourth, while inhaling, and keeping your hands where they were on the floor (if they weren't on the floor, bend your knees and place them where you wish you could have put them earlier), put your right leg back behind you, and bend the left knee until the left shin is straight up and down, and the left knee is in your armpit. Arch your back and neck until you are gazing up at the ceiling/sky. Five seconds there.

Fifth, while exhaling, put the front leg back with the back leg and point your hips and buttocks up at the ceiling (sky). Ideally, your knees and back are straight, your hands are flat on the floor at about shoulder width, and your head is in line with your torso. If you can keep your feet flat on the floor, hooray, but don't strain to get there. Hold that pose and that non-breath for the usual five seconds. This pose is called mountain pose.

The sixth begins a series of two positions that are performed in a continuous, smooth motion. The sixth is performed with the breath still inhaled. In this position you "collapse" that mountain pose, bringing your torso down closer to the floor, briefly putting your whole weight on your toes and hands, with your knees, chest and chin lightly touching the floor. Your hips don't touch the floor, and you don't stay here long, merely passing through this position on the way to:

Seven, called the "cobra" position, which is where you inhale, and with the toes, knees and hands touching the ground, arc the neck and spine back up, while you gaze upwards gaze at the ceiling. Five seconds. If any of this is difficult, just do your best. You'll eventually be able to do this well, subject, of course, to the emergence of joint flexibility and stamina, over time.

Eight, exhale, and recreate that mountain position (see number five). This and every position to follow is held for five seconds.

Nine, inhale, step forward with your left leg and put your hands down beside your foot, recreating position number four.

Ten, exhale, bring the right foot forward up by the left and redo number three.

Eleven, inhale and lean over backwards, just like you did back in number two.

Exhale while straightening up and you are back to position number one. Hold for five.

That was one set. To do another set, you start immediately start over with five seconds of the same position that you ended with.

You may have noticed that the legs don't do the same exercise in this formula, so what we do is, in the next surya, put the other leg back in step number 4 and reverse in step number nine. A balanced exercise regimen would, therefore consist of even numbers of suryanamaskars.

After you have done your set of suryas, lie down on your back to rest for a minute or so.

The thing about this and all forms of exercise, according to Maharishi Vedic Medicine, is not to strain. You don't want to push the body to extremes such that you are breathing heavily and sweating profusely. As a matter of fact, the MVM guidelines on exercise are distinctly different from what you may have received in high school gym class.

First of all, MVM suggests that you exercise less strenuously, but more often. If you can probably run a mile, run a half mile. If you can probably take a brisk walk for ten minutes, take it for five. This should be easier for you, but do it often, that is, every day.

Other exercise do's and don'ts include:

Wait to exercise for two hours after a full meal, and also wait for at least a half-hour after exercising to start a meal.

Don't strain. If your breathing gets so heavy that you have to breathe through the mouth, rather than comfortably through the nose, cut back a bit, and try again tomorrow, gradually building up to the level that you were trying to achieve. Another indication to slow down is if you start perspiring. This is the no sweat plan. Regular exercise will enable you to do more than pushing hard for a few times and then quitting.

You'll know if you are doing this right if you feel invigorated rather than fatigued at the end of your exercise session.

The best time to exercise, as we mention earlier, is from six to ten in the morning. Doing the Transcendental Meditation Program then exercise is best. The only exceptions to this are the suryas and the yoga asanas that I described above, which have the effect of settling the mind, body and breath before meditation. Surya first, then asanas, then TM.

If you are under 25 you need more exercise than those over 25, and the optimal intensity of your exercise also varies, depending on your doshic makeup. (see chart below for an initial determination of your basic dosha type)

Vata types should engage in slow-paced, light exercise that keeps the body in continuous motion for 15 to 20 minutes. You might try walking, swimming, yoga exercises and light bicycling. None of this Tour de France stuff.

Pitta types can try brisker exercises that keep them in motion for about the same amount of time, including brisk walking, moderate cross-country skiing, cycling, swimming, weight lifting, racquetball, and tennis.

Kapha types (remember, this is healthy kapha types, you are going to have to scale it down to size for a while, but this gives you a picture of where you should be) should be doing 15 to 30 minutes of vigorous exercise. This may include jogging, vigorous bicycling (parlez-vous Francais?), cross-country skiing, aerobics, walking (uphill?) and heavy weightlifting.

All three doshas can benefit from walking and from suryanamaskar, neuromuscular integration (asanas) and neurorespiratory integration exercises (more on that next). It's just that kapha people should walk a little faster, or even jog, while vatas might do well to stroll.

The chronically fatigued should start somewhere, realizing that you probably have a lot of kapha to move out. Your MVM physician will guide you. For CFS patients, even 25 steps is a start. You can do more tomorrow. But do it, and do a bit more daily.

Identifying your personal characteristics on the following chart will aid you in determining which dosha is predominant in your physiology:

Vata	Pitta	Kapha
Light build	strong hunger	solid, powerful build
Acts quickly	strong thirst	great strength
Irregular hunger	strong digestion	endurance
Irregular digestion	stress creates anger	steady energy
Light sleep	fair or ruddy skin	slow, graceful action
Interrupted sleep	dislike hot weather	tranquil, relaxed
Insomnia	enterprising	slow to anger
Enthusiastic	sharp intellect	cool, smooth skin
Vivacious	precise speech	thick, oily, pale skin
Imaginative	articulate	slow to learn
Excitable	can't skip meals	slow to forget
Changeable moods	blond hair	heavy sleepers
Learn quickly	light brown hair	slow digestion
Forget quickly	red hair	mild hunger
Worriers	live by their watch	affectionate, tolerant, forgiving
Constipation	wake up at night	can be possessive
Easily tired	Take command	slow decisions
Overexert easily	Sometimes critical	wake up slowly
Energy in spurts	determined walk	respect feelings
Hungry anytime		food brings comfort
Love change		large, liquid eyes
Irregular habits		

You probably will have a combination of those factors, but you most likely will have a predominance of one or the other, although a balanced representation of all three is also considered normal.

Back to what's good for you, no matter what dosha you are.

There is also a breathing exercise, termed the neurorespiratory integration program or pranayama. This breathing exercise is settling to vata, which is probably deeply involved in any case involving fatigue. This is used just before the Transcendental Meditation

Program, for about 5 minutes each time. This exercise balances vata dosha, cultures the mind, quiets the physiology, and serves as a calming, settling activity just before the morning and evening meditation period.

You do this practice without engaging in other activities, such as listening to the radio, watching TV or reading. Having your eyes closed helps. To do it, you sit erect, comfortably. Then, using the thumb of your right hand, you close the right nostril and breathe out of the left nostril slowly and completely. Then you gently breathe in through the left nostril, and when you have taken that inward breath, close the left nostril with your ring and middle fingers. Release the pressure on the thumb, and exhale slowly and completely through the right nostril. Gently breathe in through the right nostril, and continue switching back and forth in the same pattern, for about 5 minutes.

The Biggies

This general discussion of laudable daily behaviors can be very useful to anyone interested in better health, but what about the chronically fatigued? There may be a wide variety of symptoms associated with your particular, "customized" fatigue, but most chronic fatigue patients have common threads in the fabric of their illness, in that they are suffering from digestive problems, sleep disorders, and emotional disorders such as anxiety and depression. I'm not going to discuss digestive problems in detail here, since I'll be talking about diet in detail soon, but I will address your sleep and mood problems, and what you can do about them.

Sleep disorders are very common in both chronic fatigue and CFS. It might be considered almost a truism that bad sleep would result in fatigue. Of course, it's not quite that simple, since it can be the other way around, and factors other than the quality of rest can create insomnia, oversleeping, etc.

Sleep disorders generally have to do with vata disorders. Sometimes there can be some associated pitta imbalance. And, of course, everyone gets into the act, because increased vata and aggravated pitta vitiates (worsens) kapha, which results in sleep disorders. With kapha problems you lack calm, and can't feel settled.

Of course we are going to treat the vata imbalances via diet and panchakarma (see upcoming chapter), but we are still discussing daily routine, and we need to look at the things that you can do on your own to help alleviate these patterns.

I'm going to guess that you have one or more of the following situations: mental and/or emotional stress, excessive mental or physical activity in the evening, associated pains from any of those items in the body, muscle pain, headaches, gas pain, or poor digestion.

We will take steps to improve your digestion (later), but you can start working on reducing mental and emotional stress, if you have any control over the situation(s). You can also start de-emphasizing evening work. Think of the evening as a time to unwind rather than a time to rev up.

You need to start maintaining a strict daily routine, which should include an early, light dinner, an evening walk, if possible, and an early bedtime. We have already explained that you can also bless yourself with the Transcendental Meditation Program and yoga asanas, twice daily.

We're going to suggest that you begin listening to Gandharva Veda audio tapes. These ancient melodies are said to neutralize stress and fatigue by attuning your physiology to the cycles of nature that underly each hour of the day and each season of the year. Attuning yourself what amounts to the quantum mechanical wave function or vibrational quality of each hour as it passes begins to reset your physiology in tune with more natural daily rhythms. Sounds like a good start. [21]

We're even going to suggest that you move somewhere else from where you live right now, that you build a new home, or rent a completely different place, anyway.

No kidding, your home environment may be inhibiting your sleep. I'll be discussing this in detail later, but for now, it should be obvious that there are sick buildings just like there are sick people.

Maharishi Sthapatyaved, the science of "place," exists to guide you in choosing and living in a home that is optimized to support your greatest health and happiness. We know it's a radical prescription to tell you to move somewhere else, but there's no reason not to tell you

---

21. Maharishi University of Management Press (1-800-831-6523) has CD's that provide 24 hours of blissful Gandharva music.

the whole truth of the matter, and there's every indication that the health of many people is as if swimming upstream against the weight of the deadening environments in which they live and work.

You should also consult with an expert in Maharishi Jyotish, which is the science of you and your "cosmic counterparts," or the relationship of your individual experience to the positions of the planets in the solar system around you.

There will be more on this later, too, but for now you should know that Maharishi Jyotish is deeper than you may think, and probably like no astrological schema you've ever heard of, because it's not about fate, but rather about heyam dukham anagutam, i.e., averting the danger that has not come. That's right, there are even a set of Maharishi Yagyas, or performances, designed to neutralize negative trends in your life before they happen (or even if they are already happening) and strengthen powerful aspects.

On a practical level, and at little or no cost, you can also start engaging in the following behaviors:

- Spend time with uplifting, positive people
- Avoid smoking
- Avoid alcohol
- Avoid sleeping late (past six, remember)
- Avoid sleeping during the day
- Have some warm milk for dinner or at bedtime (boil it, then let it cool a bit), adding some nutmeg or saffron

- Do an abhyanga at 5 p.m. or so, before dinner
- Reduce evening activities
- Take an evening walk

Maharishi Vedic Medicine specifies a number of prescription and non-prescription herbal remedies, tablets, teas, decoctions and even nasally administered oils to address sleep disorders. Your MVM physician will suggest the personalized, dosha-specific versions, but even now you can benefit from generalized herbal remedies such as Slumbertime tea, Blissful Sleep tablets, Slumbertime aroma oil, Fatigue Free tablets, Worry Free tea and tablets, etc.[22]

One more thing: a nice, relaxing bath, just before bed. Not too hot, not too cold. Enjoy.

There is also hope for people that whose life experience is held in the grip of anxiety and/or depression, or emotional disorders.

These imbalances can be both causes and effects of chronic fatigue. All three doshas can be involved, although anxiety is usually caused by vata or vata/pitta imbalances. Depression is normally brought about by too much vata, kapha, or an overabundant combination of the two.

Again, we are going to focus on removing the underlying causes, through panchakarma and herbal means, plus by removing illusory effects of pragyaparadh through the Transcendental Meditation

---

22. Catalog and phone ordering available from Maharishi Ayurvedic Products International, 1-800-255-8332, or online at www.mapi.com

Program, which will automatically start bringing your activity more in tune with the natural laws of the universe.

Even so, despite the application of all those treatment modules, there is a lot that you can start doing or undoing on your own.

First of all, you will work on your daily routine, setting up a regular schedule: regular bowel movements, regular meals, and a regular bedtime.

It would be good, and soothing, for depressed and anxious people to get up early and take an early morning walk, preferably a "nature walk" in beautiful, serene surroundings. Try this tomorrow (why wait?).

You should have a purpose to your daily activities, engaging in purposeful and entertaining activities.

It's great if you can engage in healthy, uplifting activities like gardening, and playing with children. It's also wonderful if you can fill your rooms with the aroma of fresh flowers, or other aromas such as those available through MAPI (www.mapi.com). You should take steps to make sure that you inhabit and work (if possible) in an orderly, clean environment. You should bathe daily, too, and take time to enjoy it.

You need to avoid factors that create indigestion (irregular meals, eating too fast/slow, drinking too much fluids, cold/frozen foods, eating between meals, eating leftover foods, very oily food, overly spicy food, meat products, root vegetables and beans, any heavy foods). More on diet soon.

There is an array of herbs, oils and teas for these imbalances available trough MAPI, such as the Worry Free and Blissful Joy products.

There is no time like the present for getting some help.

Basically, we are going to suggest that you make use of all of the approaches of Maharishi Vedic medicine, quit smoking and drinking, or at least reduce consumption, and start digging out of that hole, with a hand to help lift you up to the light of day from this timeless knowledge of who you really are.

We should also mention that if it so happens that you are a woman, (multiple studies indicated that the majority of people receiving care for CFS are female).[23] You should rest more during menstruation. If you are pushing your way through your period without giving your body it's due, you are not really listening to your body. Among those women actively involved in the use of Maharishi Vedic medicine, the usual term for menstruation is "resting." It is wise to apply that particular euphemism on the behavioral level.

In addition to these specific bits of advice, the ancient literature mentions some general guidelines for behavior, encouraging us all to be:

- Truthful
- Free from anger

---

23. Fitzgibbon EJ, Murphy D, O'Shea K, Kelleher C, 1997, Chronic Debilitating Fatigue in Irish General Practice: A survey of General Practitioner's Experience, British Journal of General Practice, 47 (423): 618-622

- Non-indulgent in alcohol
- Non-indulgent in inappropriate sexual intercourse
- Non-overindulgent in sexual intercourse
- Non-violent
- Non-exerting
- Calm
- Sweet Spoken
- Engaged in Meditation
- Engaged in cleanliness
- Perseverant
- Observing charity
- Practicing religion
- Respectful towards teachers, preceptors and elders
- Devoted to love and compassion
- Balanced in sleep and wakefulness
- Using ghee (clarified butter) regularly
- Knowing the measure of time and place with propriety
- Unconceited
- Well-behaved
- Simple
- Controlling the senses
- Keeping the company of elders
- Positive
- Self-controlled

Devoted to scripture so, we've looked at some changes to your schedule, suggested some new behaviors, such as oil massage and some light exercise, and even added some attitude adjustments to the mix. We haven't discussed diet yet, but we will, soon enough.

One final point is the importance of your intention or will power. No application of healing forces is going to take effect without your committed involvement. You may not feel powerful. You may feel listless, or even apathetic and exhausted. But on some level you have to make a choice to come out of the cloud, even if you feel powerless to move on your own. The mental decision is the first step.

The other odd thing is that you have to start putting attention on yourself. We are nearing the close of a long chapter on how your personal behavior can change your health, on how you can change the direction of your life into a positive one. Many people would prefer to just take a pill, if it was possible, and not just because it is easier, but because they are out of the habit of caring for themselves.

When the building starts slowly falling down, the residents run out and inspect the foundation. If your fundamental behavior is not supporting health, no amount of plastering and shoring up is going to help you. This is a great time to be what many of us might consider "selfish," in that you have to start taking care of yourself.

From one perspective, you might consider that this is truly your fundamental task on this planet. The ancient Greek maxim to "know thyself" is not simply applicable to the mind. You need to take responsibility for yourself. You need to know your limitations and your strengths. When you take good care of one person in the world, i.e.- yourself, you take one person off of the list that society has to support. You also start to support others better, automatically, because with more strength, you have more to give, and with more freshness and intelligence available for your work and your life in general, you naturally contribute more to society.

If you create peace in your own heart and reduce the stress and anxiety at home, you have brought peace to the fundamental unit of world peace.

You do your personal house cleaning first, and the world gets purified.

Cleaning up can be easy, too, since hundreds of herbal and physiological aids stand ready to help you. An entire network of physicians and in-residence programs are already in place to help bring you back to health. But only you can decide to take charge of your eating habits, your daily routine, and your investment in consciousness through the Transcendental Meditation Program and the other modalities of Maharishi Vedic Medicine.

You just have to put your life in tune with natural law for a while, at least on the level of behavior, and then you will start to experience the support of nature. But as you begin taking steps in a healthy direction, health moves toward you to close the gap. The trip back to health is not a long one, since it is just rediscovering your own, vital essential nature. But you have to start the process, and maintain vigilance, and then the rest is automatic due to the application of Maharishi Vedic Medicine.

The main mechanism of all this, again, is memory. Remembering who you are. An improved routine settles your life, brings order into your world. Knowing how to integrate your living habits with the structures of nature brings your life more into tune with the laws of nature that are all around you. When you live more in tune with the laws of nature, nature is said to be more supportive of you.

In other words, when you live right, you feel right.

When you live more in tune with the rhythms of nature, the clear still note of what you are becomes more apparent, and instead of a tired bleat, your life becomes more of a song.

But first your instrument may need some cleaning.

CHAPTER 9

Rejuvenating Tired Cells

I have talked a lot about how ama gets generated inside your body, and its role in chronic fatigue, and now it's time to talk about moving the ama out of the body. One of the most effective treatments for eliminating ama at a deep level, and at the same time rekindling agni, the digestive fire, is Maharishi Rejuvenation Therapy. This therapy includes simple, natural purification treatments such as steam baths, oleation therapy, ayurvedic massage, and eliminative therapies offered at luxurious outpatient and inpatient facilities throughout the United States, Canada, and in Europe. Maharishi Rejuvenation Therapy is extremely effective in bringing balance to the doshas, and in improving overall health and eliminating chronic fatigue. Just one week of this remarkable treatment can bring stunning results.

Case Study

"Mary is a senior vice-president for a clearing firm for professional traders in Chicago. Seven years ago she was diagnosed with chronic fatigue syndrome. "I had a flu and cold that kept coming back. I was dragging to work - that's all I could do. Weekends I would spend resting so I could go back to work on Monday. By Wednesday I was thoroughly exhausted again. My life became very limited."

When her doctor told her there was nothing that she could do to alleviate the symptoms, Mary decided to take her own steps. She began reading books from her local health food store and stopped drinking alcohol and coffee, avoided sugar and took vitamins. Her condition continued.

Her first signs of improvement came when she began to investigate alternative health modalities. Acupuncture and herbs provided some relief from the constant flu and colds. After seeing a clinical nutritionist and participating in a six-month detoxification program her energy levels improved. She learned biofeedback and meditation which provided great relief. Yet several years later she still suffered periods of fatigue, and, was almost bedridden by PMS; she lived a restricted lifestyle centered around getting and staying rested.

In 1996, a bacteria picked up in a spa in Jamaica reversed some of the progress that had been made. "I couldn't get better," recalls Mary. "My digestion was out of whack and I was extremely fatigued. At that time I read a book on Ayur-Veda and had a strong feeling that I should do this."

After the initial constulation, her response was," "I thought I was doing great things for myself by eating a healthy diet. And it was healthy - but not for me. It was very much the wrong diet for me. That's what I like the best about Ayur-veda. The recommendations are so specific for your needs."

On my recommendations, Mary called one of the U.S. facilities.

Mary called one of the U.S. facilities for in-residence Maharishi Rejuvenation Therapy and immediately booked a six-day rejuvenation package. "As soon as I walked in the door I had a feeling of relaxation and comfort."

After six days of treatments and knowledge classes, Mary returned to Chicago transformed. "The results were instantaneous. I had a significant increase in energy. I have not been sick since that first visit over a year ago. Of course I continue the routine at home that I was taught, of which meditation is an important part. The doctor also gave me herbs for digestion and to boost my immune system. I can tell when I go off my diet and routine; my digestion changes and I start feeling fatigued. But I know how to get back on track. In other words, now I can control my health."

What a Treatment Is Like

If you have ever been to a health spa or had a colonic, you may think you know what I'm describing here. There may be some superficial similarities, but you cannot truly fathom the depth and sophistication of these methods until you try them.

Let's say that you have been struggling through the past few months, trying to keep up with work and home responsibilities without collapsing. Your first treatment, which is several hours long, consists of lying on a table being gently massaged by two technicians who are trained in the science of ayurvedic massage. They work in synchrony, using herbalized oils that have been chosen especially for your doshic imbalances. The oil is warm and soothing, the massage seems to rejuvenate your cells. For the first time in months, you start to feel your body's inner intelligence flowing through and nourishing your body.

One of the treatments, shirodhara, consists of warm oil being drizzled on your forehead in a specific pattern. Sounds simple, but it has a profound effect on the neurophysiology, relaxing the nervous system, synchronizing the brain waves, and balancing vata dosha. Afterwards, you feel like your brain has had a bath.

Other treatments include elimination therapies (more gentle and natural than a colonic), swedana (steam therapy) and nasya (steam and herbal therapies to cleanse the nasal passages and channels to the brain).

After the treatment, assuming you are taking the in-residence treatments, you eat prepared meals that are designed to help your digestion purify. You rest in rooms filled with aromas that are designed to balance your specific doshas. That night you sleep better than you have in years. Throughout the next few days, you can feel the stress literally being drained out of your body. You feel like you're enveloped in a warm, nourishing cocoon, that everything in your environment is nourishing, rejuvenating, and purifying you. And you are right to feel that way.

By the end of the week, you've experienced a major shift in your mind and body. You may still have a ways to go on the path to recovery, but you're no longer the victim of chronic fatigue. Your body is not the same body that you came in with. You now feel energy flowing through your body but at the same time you feel so much calmer. You feel like you can continue on the path of good health that you've started on. You return home with a home-care program that includes specific recommendations for your doshic imbalances, including simple, natural ways to change your lifestyle, diet, and exercise programs to support energy rather than fatigue.

One client said, "I don't feel like I've been rejuvenated, I feel like I've been rebuilt."

Cellular Rejuvenation

One of the reasons people feel like they have a new body after Maharishi Rejuvenation Therapy is because, in part, they do. At least they have replaced many of the toxin-filled molecules that make up their cell walls with new, fresh ones. This may sound like magic, but in fact, it's true.

The reason for this is that the cell walls are made of lipids (fats) and proteins.

The herbalized oils (also lipids) used externally in the panchakarma treatments penetrate the skin and reach its deepest layers. The new lipid molecules reach the cellular level and replace the tired, toxin-filled lipid molecules.

The result is that you feel fresher and toxins are removed at the cellular level.

The Five Actions of Panchakarma

At the core of Maharishi Rejuvenation Therapy is a series of purification procedures called panchakarma, which means "five actions." In general, the ayurvedic strategy is to liquefy ama and balance doshas and get rid of toxins through the elimination system. Through this purification process, the srotas are cleared and doshas are balanced. Then the body is more receptive to treatment, such as rasayanas and herbal formulas.

The five actions of panchakarma, which include snehana (internal purification with oils) swedana (steam therapy) and abhyanga (oil massage) and nasya(nasal therapy) and basti (herbalized enemas) are all part of the field of internal medicine known as kayachikitsa.

Kayachikitsa is concerned with balancing the internal digestive fire, which is exactly what is needed in treating chronic fatigue.

Here's a description of the treatments included in Maharishi Rejuvenation Therapy.

Internal Purification Therapy (Snehana)

Snehana is an important part of Maharishi Rejuvenation Therapy, and it begins a week before the other treatments. While still at home, the patient takes a measure of ghee or herbal tea each day for five days.

This treatment is designed to loosen up and soften hardened impurities, allowing them to pass into the digestive system and out of the body through its normal elimination process. The ghee goes through the digestive system quickly, penetrates the body's lipid cell walls and loosens the impurities. The herbal version has a similar effect.

Laxative Therapy (Virechena)

Once the impurities--which have been loosened by snehana-- start to move into the digestive tract, it's important to eliminate them from the body efficiently. For this, a mild laxative therapy is employed, called virechana. Virechana is gentle yet effective in cleansing impurities from the intestines, and is an important part of the purification process. It is especially useful for eliminating excessive Pitta and Kapha doshas from the body. Virechena is usually done after snehana and before the other treatments begin.

Basically we've loosened up the bad stuff and then we're cleaning it out. This is before you even get started with all the massage stuff. Just doing this part can already give you a sense of rejuvenation.

Another elimination therapy, used throughout the treatments described below, is called basti. Bastis are essentially herbal enemas, and they can be formulated either for purification or nourishment. They gently remove impurities and normalize vata, which is seated in the large intestine. This is an important therapy in eliminating Chronic Fatigue, because it balances the digestive and elimination systems, and is used to treat constipation, abdominal disorders, loss of strength, fatigue, diarrhea, chest pain, spleen disorders, fever, headache, earache, backache, stiffness, and other problems caused by an out of balance vata dosha.

Massage Therapies

There are a number of massage therapies, and each has a specific purpose in balancing the doshas.

Abhyanga

Abhyanga, or ayurvedic oil massage, is the most common massage therapy used in Maharishi Rejuveantation Therapy. You already learned how to do abhyanga in the chapter on the daily routine. The procedure is similar, except that here there are two trained technicians, one on each side of the body, to administer the massage in a kind of synchronized motion. You can imagine that this will be even easier than that easy self-treatment. Plus, these guys are pros (or ladies for female patients) It also lasts much longer, up to an hour.

This balanced massage actually integrates the two hemispheres of your brain, creating a balanced, integrated experience.

Luxurious and relaxing, abhyanga is designed to stimulate what are termed the marma points of the body, which Maharishi Vedic Medicine describes as are the junction points between consciousness and matter, or the "switchboards" that control a section of the nervous system.

Abhyanga also balances vata dosha, the "king" dosha that leads the others, and is a major factor in most Chronic Fatigue patients.

Abhyanga also purifies the body by moving impurities, which have been loosened by snehana, into the bloodstream and digestive tract to be eliminated easily from the body. More loosening and more letting go of the bad stuff.

Oils used in Abhyanga

The sesame oil used in abhyanga contains herbs to balance vata, pitta, or kapha dosha, depending on the patient's needs.

In the case of patients with Chronic Fatigue or other chronic illness, special herb and oil mixtures, some containing up to 75 herbs, may be prescribed that remove physiological weakness by purifying the dhatus (tissues).

Traditionally, sesame oil is recommended for most panchakarma treatments, because it balances vata dosha and has a soothing, nourishing effect on the mind and body.

Research shows that sesame oil has an anti-bacterial effect when used daily on the skin. This may be because sesame oil is composed of 40% linoleic acid, which is known to inhibit growth of bacteria and is a powerful anti-inflammatory agent.

In further research, Drs. Edwards Smith and John Salerno found that sesame oil appears to be anticarcinogenic. Of course other oils may be prescribed for particular needs.

Nasya

Nasya is a technique to clear impurities from the head, ears, and sinuses. Part of the treatment involves inhaling herbalized steam through the nose, which helps clear out mucus from the lungs and nasal passages. This effect is furthered by installation of various herbal drops in the nose. This treatment is especially beneficial for people who suffer from hay fever, headache, earache, lung diseases, tonsillitis, or weakened lungs. It also creates better mind body coordination, stimulating the base of the brain and creating balance in the mind, brain, senses and thyroid gland.

Udvartana

This is a massage designed to balance kapha dosha, cleanse the skin, increase blood circulation to deeper tissues, and promote weight loss. Instead of using sesame oil, this massage uses a paste of rice and other grains. It is stimulating rather than relaxing. Some of you may need stimulating. Your physician will know best.

Garshan

This is another massage that stimulates circulation, removes impurities, and is useful in treating weight problems and cellulite.

Instead of using sesame oil, the massage technician uses wool or raw silk gloves to stimulate the skin.

Heat Treatments ("fomentation")

Heat is an important element in Maharishi Rejuvenation therapy, because the impurities need to be heated, liquefied, and passed out of the body. Heat dilates the body's channels, allowing the impurities to pass through easily, and it softens impurities that have become hardened. Heat treatments are especially helpful for treating muscle, joint, and bone problems, and Vata and Kapha disorders such as Chronic Fatigue.

Swedana

Swedana is basically an herbal steam bath for the whole body except the head. Swedana is a very effective therapy, allowing impurities to be eliminated through sweat glands. Swedana is useful in balancing Vata and Kapha disorders, and is used to treat constipation, asthma, arthritis, and paralysis.

Pizzichilli

This heat treatment is also a massage, and probably the most luxurious and relaxing experience you'll ever have. While two technicians massage the body, herbalized oil is poured over the body in a constant stream while the massage is going on. It feels like an oil bath. The constant flow of oil penetrates the deepest layers of the tissues, repairing deep imbalances in the musculoskeletal system. It also pacifies the cold and dry vata dosha.

Pinda Swedana

This is another heat treatment that is also a massage. It uses cloth pillows filled with a warm mixture of rice, herbs and milk to massage the body. This heat treatment increases nourishment, strength and balance, especially to the joints and neuromuscular system.

Shirodhara and Netra Tarpana

There are several other treatments that are an important part of Maharishi Rejuvenation Therapy. These include shirodhara, mentioned above, which creates deep relaxation, brain-wave coherence, and profound mental rest. It is an important treatment for people with Chronic Fatigue, because it deeply relaxes the nervous system and provides deep rest.

Netra tarpana is a treatment that cleanses the eyes with ghee and herbal smoke, removing eye strain.

Aroma Therapy

While resting after treatment, you will be treated to one of the most enjoyable of all the therapies of Maharishi Vedic Medicine Maharishi aroma therapy. Maharishi aroma therapy uses herb and flower extracts to balance the doshas. Like the herbal compounds of Maharishi Vedic Medicine, Maharishi Aroma Therapy does not use single herbs. Rather, it uses a combination of extracts to create a holistic, balanced effect on the doshas.

Smell is one of the most powerful of the senses, because it is associated with the limbic area of the brain, linked with both emotions and memory. It's also one of the easiest therapies to use, because you can use it while you sleep, or in the office while you're working. The aromas are also extremely pleasant. You can use an aroma pot or an aroma diffuser that fits into a wall socket to dispense the aromas.

Besides vata, pitta, and kapha aroma formulas, many other aroma mixtures are available. One of the most important for Chronic Fatigue patients is an aroma blend that contains a balanced blend of essential oils- juniper berry, patchouli, jasmine, and others to help boost energy levels. There are several other fatigue-related aroma blends that may be of help as well. All available at the Health and Wholeness stores, or at www.mapi.com.

Clearing the Srotas on a Seasonal Basis

One of the main beneficial effects of Maharishi Rejuvenation Therapy is to clear obstructions from the srotas, a process called srota shuddhi. Once the srotas are cleared, the body's own repair mechanisms can function again, allowing the body to heal and restore its natural balance.

Also, once the channels are cleared that carry rasa (nutritional fluids), the tired cells that have been deprived of nutrition can regenerate themselves, resulting in renewed energy and vigor. Finally, the srotas that remove waste from the body, once cleared, can more easily do their job to ensure that toxins no longer build up.

The effects of Maharishi Rejuvenation Therapy are profound and long-lasting. However, over time, seasonal changes and the stress of modern life can cause the same build-up of toxins and blockage to the srotas to happen again, although to a lesser degree.

That is why the ancient texts recommend having Maharishi Rejuvenation therapy on a seasonal basis. The doshas tend to build up and become aggravated during one season, and it is healthy to cleanse the body of the excess doshas and toxins before the new season starts. This is the ideal schedule for maintaining health and vitality all year round, and it is the ideal way to prevent disease or fatigue from cropping up.

Clearing the srotas is the best preparation for taking rasayanas (more on these beneficial herbal elixirs later) and other herbal food supplements. Then the rasayanas and herbal preparations can easily reach their targeted cells, repairing and reminding the body of the memory of wholeness and proper functioning.

Research on Maharishi Rejuvenation Therapy

Since the mid 1980s, when Maharishi Rejuvenation Therapy began to be offered in the United States and other countries in the West, thousands of people have enjoyed the profoundly rejuvenating results of these treatments.

For people suffering from Chronic Fatigue, the results are promising. Research published in the Journal of social Behavior and Personality has found that Maharishi Rejuvenation Therapy improves vitality, energy, appetite and digestion, clarity of mind, a general sense of well-being, and gives relief from various health problems.[24]

Additional research also indicates that fatigue can be helped by these therapies. A study showed statistically significant declines in unhealthy emotional states such as anxiety, depression, fatigue, and confusionand increased energy.[25]

Drs. Robert Herron and John Fagen have shown that these therapies greatly reduce the levels of fourteen important lipophilic (fat soluable) toxic and carcinogenic chemicals in the body. These toxins

24. The Journal of Social Behavior and Personality, vol. 5 (1990), pp. 1-27
25. Data presented at the International College of Psychosomatic Medicine, Eighth World Congress, Chicago, Illinois, 1985. Improvements in Health with the Maharishi Ayurveda Program; Journal of Social Behavior and Personality 5 (1990), pp. 1-27.

cause immune system suppression, hormone disruption, reproductive disorders and cancers. Another study found significant imporovement in cardoivscular risk factors by these therapies.

All in all, I think that you might enjoy this treatment. It will certainly be memorable, as it enlivens your memory of who you really are.

CHAPTER 10

Herbs and Food Supplements for Vitality

We've talked about you for a while, Now let's consider Nancy, a working mother with two young children and a stressful job who came to my office with complaints of debilitating migraines, PMS, insomnia, digestive problems, and extreme fatigue. Sound familiar?

She had seen several physicians and had a thorough work-up of tests for her symptoms, but the tests revealed no causes. Thoroughly disillusioned, she had turned to few alternative remedies with equally depressing results.

Literally in tears, she told me that she could no longer handle her responsibilities. "Why haven't these helped?" she asked, gesturing to a grocery bag of vitamins, minerals, and herbal remedies that she was now taking and had brought to show me.

To answer Nancy, I had to explain several principles of the science of dravayaguna, or ayurvedic herbal formulas for healing. This ancient science of preparing herbs is highly sophisticated, and involves methods and techniques that are unknown in Western herbal preparation.

First of all, the vitamins and commercially-prepared herbs that Nancy was taking did not address the root cause of her problem, namely ama and an underlying imbalance in the doshas created by irregular eating habits, irregular routine, and mental pressure. Bad habits were shutting down her digestion, causing ama to accumulate, and creating tired, toxin-filled cells.

She needed to take herbal formulas that specifically improved digestion and removed impurities as well as targeting her specific doshic imbalances (which in this case was vata dosha). She also needed to make some changes in lifestyle, diet, and stress reduction in order to pave the way for the effectiveness of the herbal formulas. Just like most chronically fatigued people.

I also pointed out that most commercial vitamins are synthetically made, and are so concentrated as to tax the liver, which is often already overloaded in patients with chronic fatigue. Maharishi Vedic Medicine recommends that people get their supply of vitamins from eating whole foods, i.e. - whole fruits and vegetables. Once the body is purified of excess toxins and ama, most people can get their nutritional needs through food alone.

It often becomes a vicious cycle, as the patient with Chronic Fatigue takes commercial vitamins in an attempt to gain energy and is prescribed allopathic medication for various symptoms. And both vitamins and medications are constipating, throwing the digestion further off balance.

The commercial herbal preparations that Nancy bought at the health food store typically used the allopathic technique of isolating and extracting the active ingredient to "enhance" the power of the herb. Unfortunately, herbal formulas composed of such active ingredients can actually create harmful side-effects, similar to (but not as powerful as) those created by allopathic drugs.

In Maharishi Ayur-Veda, on the other hand, the whole herb is crushed and added to the formula rather than just the active ingredient. This ensures the inclusion of the naturally designed balancing agents that the herb contains.

Rather than using the harmful and unnatural technique of extracting the active ingredient, the Vedic texts explain in detail how to increase the power of the main herb by combining it with other herbs, chosen especially for their enhancing qualities.

Many of the bottles in Nancy's bag contained single herbs. You will almost never find single herbs used in Maharishi Ayur-Veda, but rather will find them mixed together in herbal formulas. By combining the herbs in these traditional formulas, the healing power of individual herbs is increased and side effects that might be created by a single herb are softened and eliminated.

Maharishi Ayur-Vedic formulas do, however, usually start with a main ingredient, an herb to treat fatigue, for instance. Herbs with similar properties and healing effects are then added to support the main herb.

When you combine certain herbs together in a formula, you create an effect that is more powerful than the effects of the single herbs. The synergistic effect of combining several herbs that treat fatigue will be more powerful, and create a broader-spectrum effect than the same amount of a single herb.

Besides the main healing herbs, there will also be herbs added to cure secondary effects. For instance, in treating fatigue, additional herbs will be added to clear the circulatory channels, stimulate the digestion, and increase resilience to stress, since these all are related to fatigue. These secondary herbs broaden the effect of the formula and make it more holistic.

Third, some herbs will be added that actually have the opposite effect than the main herbs. The reason for this is simple: to create more balance and prevent too strong a reaction. This is how harmful side-effects are avoided. Spicy herbs might be balanced by the addition of raw sugar; drying herbs will be balanced with the addition of ghee. This also makes the herbs more palatable.

Other herbs will be added to increase absorption or digestibility by the body. Some formulas contain as many as five herbs for this purpose.

All Maharishi Ayur-Veda herbal formulas also include herbs to detoxify the channels (srotas) of the body, since the herbs cannot even reach their target cells if the srotas are blocked. These herbs sometimes work as a laxative, supporting the body's elimination system as well.

Finally, an "anupam" ingredient is included that helps carry the herbs to the deep tissues and to the cells themselves. Honey, ghee, and milk are common carriers. These ensure that the herbs actually reach their target.

You can see how these ancient herbal formulas can be much more powerful, highly sophisticated, yet safer than taking active ingredient-based single herbal and medicinal formulas.

The Vedic texts are remarkable in their sophistication and knowledge of these effects of herb combining. It may seem mind-boggling at first glance to see how the thousands of herbs in the ayurvedic pharmacopeia can be combined to create very specific effects. Yet all of the herbal formulas are based on four principles for combining herbs: taste (rasa), energy (virya), aftertaste (vipaka), and potency (prabhava).

Taste (rasa) refers to the six tastes (described in chapter 11) --sweet, sour, salty, bitter, pungent and astringent. Herbs are classified according to these tastes in the same way as food, and they have a similar effect on the doshas. Sweet herbs, for instance, will balance Vata and Pitta doshas just as a sweet tasting food would. Sour herbs increase Pitta and Kapha. Through taste, different herbs will affect the doshas in different ways.

Energy (virya) has to do with the power or energy contained in the herbs, classified primarily according to whether they are heating or cooling and secondarily according to whether they are dry or moist. There is also the aftertaste (vipaka) has to do with the effect that the herb has after digestion. Herbs that are bitter and astringent to the taste, for instance, have a pungent post-digestive effect. The different after-tastes can thus be used in different ways, similar to the tastes, to treat digestive disorders.

The potency (prabhava) of the herb describes the more subtle, non-material properties of the herb. Some herbs may have the properties of heating, yet are known to have a cooling effect. Prabhava explains the effects on the mind and consciousness that are sometimes more subtle than the other three properties of herbs.

The Vedic texts describe many traditional methods for preparing the herbs, and all of them retain the natural properties of the whole herb. These methods include preparing fresh juices, herbal pastes, decoctions, hot infusion, cold infusion, pills and tablets, powders, jellies, medicated oils, and medicated ghees.

In all of these methods, the temperature is never raised to the point that the herb's natural properties are destroyed, which is why some herbal formulas can take several weeks to prepare.

You can see that these formulas are carefully designed to create a holistic, energizing effect on the body. Since all of the herbal formulas improve elimination and digestion, they all have the side-benefit of increasing energy, even if that is not their stated purpose. The whole body is strengthened and rejuvenated at the same time that a specific imbalance is corrected. This is a far cry from the effects created by allopathic drugs, where often the entire body is debilitated and thrown into imbalance by the effects of single ingredient drugs.

After explaining these points to Nancy, I advised her to stop taking all of the vitamins and commercial herbs that she had in her grocery bag. Instead, I prescribed a diet to reduce ama and correct her doshic imbalances, some lifestyle changes to help her get on a more regular schedule, and suggested that she start the Transcendental Meditation Program™ to reduce stress. I also prescribed some Maharishi Ayur-Veda herbal formulas to address her symptoms, improve her digestion, and help her body release the toxic load it was carrying.

Within a few weeks, she was feeling more energy. In two months, she reported that most of her symptoms were gone, and that her normal vitality and stability were restored.

There are a number of herbal formulas that are available from Maharishi Ayur-Veda stores that are of special interest to Chronic Fatigue patients.

Rasayanas

The Vedic texts describe special herbal formulas called rasayanas that promote longevity, memory, intelligence, freedom from disease, youthfulness, excellence of luster, complexion, clarity of voice, optimum strength of the body and clarity of the sense organs. These are called rasayanas, and have the effect of creating more ojas than other herbal formulas.

Rasayanas are so named because they support "rasa," which we described earlier as the nutrient fluid and first of the seven dhatus. By enhancing the nutrient fluid, rasayanas support all of the seven dhatus.

Some rasayanas are for enhancing mental acuity or memory; others are for overall immunity and for developing higher states of consciousness.

Maharishi Amrit Kalash

Maharishi Amrit Kalash is considered the "king" of ayurvedic rasayanas. It is known in the Vedic texts to be an elixir that is especially helpful in clearing away toxins and free radicals. It is a very powerful antioxidant, or scavenger (a substance that clears away free radicals).

You've probably heard of antioxidants, and maybe you've taken a few to try to gain more energy. While the theory behind taking antioxidants such as Vitamin A, E, and C is sound, in practice few of the commercial varieties will help you much because they do not penetrate to the level where free radicals are generated. In other words, they don't work.

Let's back up a moment and talk about free radicals. Free radicals are the highly reactive oxidizing molecules that cause cars to rust and organic matter to decay. In your body, they help fight infection but, when found in excess, they cause aging and ninety-percent of degenerative diseases, from atherosclerosis (hardening of the arteries) to cancer to heart disease. Free radicals are also potentially implicated in chronic fatigue, both as a cause and an effect.

Free radicals breed in excess when they have a lot of decaying material to feed on. Sound familiar? You guessed it. When toxins and ama build up in the body, free radicals are created, and when they are created in excess, they attack the body itself.

Besides following all of the recommendations presented in this book to help decrease ama, another thing you can do to decrease free radicals is take Maharishi Amrit Kalash.

Research on Maharishi Amrit Kalash indicates that it is 1000 times more effective than Vitamin C in scavenging free radicals.[26]

The reason for this may lie in the methods used to prepare Maharishi Amrit Kalash. There are more than fifty fruits and herbs that are crushed whole and prepared in a traditional process, using 225 discrete steps over a period of thirty days. The mixture is prepared with ghee as the anupanam or carrier substance.

Ghee is a lipid that can penetrate the walls of the cells. Researchers postulate that the ghee and other substances allow the herbs to move through the digestive system, reach the cells, penetrate the cell membranes, and create effects inside the cells. It is this ability to penetrate the cell that makes Maharishi Amrit Kalash much more effective than other commercial antioxidants.

Maharishi Amrit Kalash also has many other life-enhancing properties. Research shows that it helps improve general well-being, removes chemical toxicity, lowers cholesterol, reduces platelet aggregation (related to atherosclerosis), and improves immunity.

---

26. H. M. Sharma, et. al, "Inhibition of Human Low-Density Lipoprotein Oxidation in Vitro by Maharishi Amrit Kalash and Maharishi Coffee Substitute" Pharmacology, Biochemistry and Behavior, Vol. 43, (1992) pp. 1175-1182.

I highly recommend Maharishi Amrit Kalash to patients who suffer from Chronic Fatigue. Many people who take Maharishi Amrit Kalash regularly for more than a year report that they no longer get colds.

Since people with Chronic Fatigue often suffer from secondary illnesses and often contract frequent colds, flu, and other infectious disease, this is a powerful yet safe way to boost your immunity and overall well-being. It is probably the most powerful food supplement that you can take to purify your body of toxins, strengthen your digestion, and build up your strength and energy. It has the most holistic and beneficial effect on mind, body, and emotions.

INCREASED RESISTANCE TO DISEASE

Research shows that Maharishi Amrit Kalash:

- Increases immunity
- Prevents atherosclerosis by reducing human platelet aggregation
- Reduces LDL (bad) cholesterol
- Reduces chemical toxicity[27]

Energizing Fatigued Cells

You'll remember that in talking about the progression of chronic fatigue, we outlined several steps: a weak digestive fire (agni) causes

---

27. Enhanced Lymphoproliferative Response, Macrophage-Mediated Tumor Cell Killing and Nitric Oxide Production After Ingestion of an Ayurvedic Drug (Maharishi Amrit Kalash), Biochemical Archives, Vol. 9, (1993) pp. 365-374. [88]
- H.M. Sharma, et al, "Maharishi Amrit Kalash Prevents Human Platelet Aggregation," Clinica and Terapia Cardiovascolare, Vol. 8, No. 3, (1989) pp. 227-230. [88]

digestion to become irregular; poor digestion leads to imbalance in Vata and Kapha dosha; due to weak agni and Vata-Kapha imbalances, and ama starts to accumulate. We also mentioned that when ama blocks the channels (srotas) that supply nutrient fluid to the cells, the cells no longer receive the kind of nourishment that they need.

Ama can also prevent waste from being carried out of the cells by the body's natural waste-removal systems. Thus the cells actually become tired, filled with tired, old waste material, and starving for new nutrition and energy. This situation on the cellular level is experienced as fatigue on the personal level.

What is needed is rejuvenation of the body's own mechanisms for replacing tired, old cells with new ones. There are several fatigue-busting formulas mentioned in the Vedic texts, which do just this, along with removing ama and powering up agni.

Fatigue Free

Ancient Vedic texts refer to fatigue as "angamarda" and describe an herbal formula called "angamarda prashamana," which is a combination of herbs that regenerate cell growth and thus treat fatigue. In recent years this herbal formula has been recreated, using the techniques and ingredients described in the texts, and it is called Fatigue Free.

- A. N. Hanna, et al, "Effect of Herbal Mixtures MAK-4 and MAK-5 on Susceptibility of Human LDL to Oxidation, Complementary Medicine International, Vol. 3, No. 3, pp. 28-36, May/June 1996. [88]
-S. C. Bondy, et al, "Antioxidant Preperties of Two Ayurvedic Herbal Preparations (MAK-4 and MAK-5)," Biochemical Archives, Vol. 10, pp. 25-31, 1994. [88]

Fatigue Free contains Country Mallow and Winter Cherry along with minerals to help clear out accumulated impurities from the body, reversing the energy-sapping accumulation of fatigue elements in the body:

Fatigue Free helps increase the body's resilience to stress-related fatigue; boosts cell regeneration, helping the body to replace toxin-laden cells with fresh, vital ones; dissolves ama; increases the flow of healthy nutrients to the cells; and promotes overall vitality and longevity. That's a good list of stuff to get rid of along with excellent replacements for the old stuff.

Here are some of the 17 ingredients contained in Fatigue Free and their properties as described in the Vedic texts:

Country Mallow (Aala) is the leading herb in a renowned Ayurvedic energy tonic called Dashmula. Combined with nine restorative herbs, country mallow is famous for helping the body replace dead cells quickly.

Indian Goosberry (Amalaki), Indian Long Pepper (Pippali) and Winter Cherry (Ashwagandha) when combined create a rasayana that promotes overall vitality and longevity.

Licorice, nutmeg, ginger, black pepper, long pepper and greater galangal improve digestion and the flow of nutrients to the cells.

Licorice, greater galangal, nutmeg, ginger, and winter cherry also help clear impurities from the srotas (microchannels).

Winter cherry (Ashwagandha) is a powerful adaptogenic herb. It helps the body adapt to and recover from stress.

Yasad Bhasma is a source of the trace mineral zinc and is valuable in fighting fatigue.

Vital Woman and Vital Man

Two other revitalizing herbal formulas are Vital Woman and Vital Man. Vital Woman helps strengthen resistance to stressful situations, balances the mind and emotions, aids natural elimination and purification of toxins from the body, helps regulate the quality and quantity of blood, and supports normal fluid balance and lubrication of the skin.

Vital Woman also helps with digestion, assimilation, and metabolism of food--to make sure the food you eat energizes your cells and in turn, energizes you.

Here are some of the 26 herbs in Vital Woman preparation:

Balya herbs for greater stamina and resistance to outside influences.

Bringhana herbs to balance the body tissues (dhatus)

Jeevanya herbs to enhance longevity and protect against premature aging. They develop the ability to look younger than your biological age--an area called Vayastag.

Prajasthapana herbs to help balance hormonal flow and strengthen the reproductive system.

Shonitasthapana herbs to help balance the quality and quantity of blood.

The care taken to produce ancient formulas such as Vital Woman is mind-boggling. The herbal source for iron in Vital Woman (Bhasma) is processed with Indian Gooseberry (Amalaki) to enhance the assimilation of iron. Just this one ingredient takes 21 steps and over a month to complete.

Vital Man enhances mental performance, the heart and emotions, purity of the blood, digestion, and fluid balance. Like the Fatigue Free formula, Vital Man includes the fatigue-busting herbs called Angamarda Prashamana. These help balance energy production and stimulates the replacement of tired, toxin-filled cells with new, energetic ones. The result is an increase in energy in your body.

Here are some of the 22 herbs in Vital Man preparation:

Winter Cherry (Ashwagandha), which nourishes the nervous system and helps calm the fight-or-flight response in a stressful situation.

Mineral Pitch (Shilajit), which helps balance the other herbs. This one ingredient takes three months to prepare.

Indian Asparagus Root, Black Musale and Licorice increase the reproductive fluid, increasing inner vitality and more energy.

Stress-Reducing Herbal Formulas

Sometimes fatigue is caused by stress. If this is the case your physician trained in Maharishi Vedic Medicine may prescribe herbal formulas such as Mind Power (to increase energy, creativity, perception, and consciousness; to increase the mental functions of acquisition, retention, and recall; to balance the emotions, increase self-confidence, and contentment; and to increase the production of ojas). Remember that ojas is the material form of consciousness in the body. If you want your body to be energetic and full of vitality, you must increase the production of ojas.

An herbal formula such as Blissful Joy may also be prescribed, especially if the fatigue is emotion-based or accompanied by depression. The herbs in Blissful Joy help balance Kapha dosha (which can bring depression when out of balance); promotes a natural zest for life; nourishes the mind-body connection and balances the emotions; improves mental functioning; aids metabolism and cell growth, which if out of balance can produce impurities that cloud the mind and emotions.

Finally, if the mental stress and anxiety is the cause of the fatigue, a formula such as Worry Free may be prescribed. Worry Free enhances the mind's natural ability to function in a calm, focused and decisive manner. It helps balance Vata dosha, especially the areas related to the brain, nervous system, breathing, circulation, and digestion; and it nourishes the mind-body connection, allowing you to respond calmly when faced with stressful situations.

I think that you'll agree that these herbs are uniquely poised to do you a lot of good. Just hearing about what they are designed to do has to be of some interest to anyone suffering from chronic fatigue, since there are so many good things covered by these formulations that some of them at least must match some if not all of your symptoms.

CHAPTER 11

Foods for Energy

John was 68, retired and single when he came to me with extreme fatigue. His medical records showed that he had a history of high blood pressure for 20 years, and had sustained a stroke three years before from which he had mostly recovered. He also had cardiac bypass surgery a few years earlier, and his heartbeat continued to be irregular. His blood pressure was very high (200/100) and his pulse rate was 98 beats per minute.

He was on several medications, including Norvasc and Zestril for high blood pressure, Lanoxin for irregular heartbeat, and Coumadin, a blood thinner. Unfortunately, the medications did not lower his blood pressure, and were causing serious side effects. He complained of dizziness, headaches, zero energy, and bloated feeling after eating. "This medicine is making me very tired and wacky," he said. "My doctors don't understand. They just tell me that I have to stay on it."

John was very tired of taking the medications that were no longer helping him. He said that with each medication he seemed to respond for a little while, and then his body would stop responding and the doctors would try a new round of medications.

After questioning him about his diet and daily routine, I found that he ate a typical bachelor's diet of canned and packaged foods. He literally ate no fresh or energizing foods at all. I explained that there was no life energy in the foods he was eating. Instead of creating energy in the body, they create more dullness and fatigue. And besides, there are many additives, and preservatives and salt which would all aggravate his blood pressure.

He was put on a simple diet of fresh vegetables, fruit, grains, and a little chicken or turkey, since he was a non-vegetarian. Exactly one month after I put him on an ayurvedic regimen of diet, herbs, and an exercise protocol of moderate walking every day, his blood pressure fell to 135 over 88. His pulse rate was 84 per minute, and there was less irregularity. "I'm getting better and I have more energy," he said at his one-month check-up. "I haven't felt this well for a very long time."

The following month his blood pressure was still only 140 over 85 and he was still feeling good despite the fact that he was only able to follow the program with about 60% of success. At this point his cardiologist took him off Zestril and reduced his Norvasc and Lanoxin to half doses. His other associated symptoms such as dizziness and headaches had almost completely disappeared. Although it was beyond the comprehension of the patient and his cardiologist, John had responded well to Maharishi Vedic Medicine.

In this case, the chronic fatigue was primarily drug-induced, and secondarily due to long-standing disease and poor dietary habits. You can see that Maharishi Vedic Medicine is perfectly compatible with conventional medicine, and it helps in reducing side effects of conventional medicine, and when used in conjunction with it, curbs imbalances and helps in reducing or eliminating unneeded medications.

Food is Energy

At the basis of everything in nature is an infinite energy field, and one of the primary ways that humans access the energy of nature is through food.

In Maharishi Vedic Medicine there is a word for this life force: prana. Food has varying amounts of prana depending on how fresh and wholesome it is. A piece of ripened fruit, picked right from the tree, would have maximum prana. That same piece of fruit eaten from a can would have zero prana. To have prana, food must be fresh.

Growing your food in the garden and picking it just before cooking would be the most ideal, but most people today don't have time for that. If you buy fresh fruits and vegetables from the grocery store and cook a batch for each meal, you are probably ingesting as much prana as possible in this modern world.

I can hear you saying, "but how can I cook fresh meals when I feel so exhausted I can barely get out of bed." But can you hear my response that eating fast foods may be at the root of your fatigue problem? If you "cook" your meals from packages, frozen foods, or cans--or if you eat a lot of leftovers--then you are not gaining any prana from your food, and you have every reason to feel tired.

Besides just eating fresh foods, there are certain foods that boost energy, and certain foods that drain it.

Energy Boosting foods

In Maharishi Vedic Medicine, certain types of foods are called "sattvic" or "pure" because they digest easily and produce more ojas. They boost energy. These include milk, lassi, ghee, olive oil, rice, wheat, barley, whole grains, freshly cooked vegetables, fresh fruits, almonds, and raw honey. These foods are light, easily digested, and also balance Vata dosha, a major player in fatigue.

Here's a word on the most important of these foods:

Milk:

These days, milk has a bad name. It's blamed for all kinds of allergies and for lactose intolerance. Yet according to Maharishi Vedic Medicine, it is one of the most important sattvic, energy-building foods because it is easily transformed into ojas. So why the discrepancy?

One reason is that the traditional texts give two suggestions for making milk more digestible that are not known in modern dietetics. First of all, milk should be boiled before you drink it. You can add a slice of fresh ginger, or a pinch of turmeric, or a pinch of cardamom. These spices and the boiling process help increase its digestibility. You can also add a little water to whole milk to make it less rich.

Secondly, milk does not combine well with salty, sour, bitter, or astringent tastes. It can actually cause gas, bloating, and other digestive problems when mixed with fruits, vegetables, meats, and fish. For this reason, it's best to drink it by itself, not with a full meal that has all those mixed tastes. Milk can be digested when it is combined with other sweet foods, such as wheat, cereals, raw sugar, and honey.

Finally, today's milk often contains the effects of additives, antibiotics, and growth hormones that have been given to the cows and that pass into the milk. They can interfere with digestion and are harmful in other ways. For this reason, it is highly recommended that you consume only organic milk and milk products.

If you still have trouble digesting milk after following all of these recommendations, special herbs for people with lactose intolerance are available at Maharishi Vedic Medical Centers.

Yogurt and lassi:

Yogurt is a milk product that is also considered sattvic, especially when diluted with water to make a pleasant drink called lassi. Lassi is the best way to have yogurt, because it is light and is not as sour. Maharishi Vedic Medicine recommends drinking it after the main meal of the day to aid digestion. It contains many digestive enzymes such as acidophilus, and has long been considered an effective digestive aid.

Curiously, yogurt gets old very quickly and therefore is best eaten freshly made. One easy way to make yogurt is to purchase a yogurt maker and follow the directions. To make yogurt on your own, boil two cups of milk with a slice of ginger. Let it cool to 110-112 F (slightly above body temperature--you can use a candy thermometer to measure) and pour into a jar. Then add half teaspoon of organic, plain yogurt per cup of milk. Set in a warmed oven overnight for six to ten hours with the oven light turned on to retain warmth, and by morning, you will have yogurt.

To make lassi, combine 1/4 c. yogurt and 3/4 c. water in a blender. Mix with a teaspoon of Rose Petal Conserve to make a refreshing and healthy drink. To make a "salty" lassi to aid digestion, add a pinch of salt and a pinch of roasted cumin seeds instead of the Rose Petal Conserve and blend.

Ghee:

Ghee is one of the most cherished and sattvic foods because it is easily converted into ojas. In fact, it shares many of the energy-giving properties of ojas itself. Vedic texts say that ghee is a stimulant for digestion, supports glow of the skin and inner beauty, enhances memory and stamina, promotes longevity and protects the body from disease.

When ghee is used for cooking the meal, or added as a flavoring, it stimulates the digestive fire. One teaspoon per meal is about right; you wouldn't want to eat more than two tablespoons of ghee maximum, as in large quantities it would increase Kapha dosha.

Ghee is mostly made up of short-chain fatty acids, which means that unlike butter and other animal fats (which are mostly made up of long-chain fatty acids), it is easily assimilated, absorbed, and then metabolized to release energy. Ghee has a balanced ratio of short-chain saturated fatty acids and monosaturated fatty acids, contains conjugated linoleic acid, a chemical thought to have anticarcinogenic properties, and has antioxidants and vitamins A, D, E, and K. Some research shows that ghee does not raise blood cholesterol levels, but until there is conclusive research, if you have high cholesterol, you should follow your doctor's advice concerning eating ghee.

Ghee is made by boiling unsalted sweet butter for about an hour. During this process, the water content boils away and the milk solids settle to the bottom and are discarded. The liquid that remains can be stored at room temperature and does not need to be refrigerated. You can also buy ghee at some stores and through www.mapi.com.

One of the best uses for ghee is as cooking oil. Ghee does not burn like other oils do when heated, and thus does not create free radicals. It is therefore ideal for sauteing spices and vegetables and also as a spread on bread instead of butter.

Dhal:

One of the most easily digested and wholesome sources of protein is dhal, or split mung beans. You can purchase this at Indian grocery stores. Dhal is made by boiling one part mung dhal per three parts water for about twenty to thirty minutes, and adding sauteed spices such as fresh ginger, cumin seed, coriander powder, turmeric, and salt. The spices also aid digestion. It's best to eat dhal with rice or another whole grain to create a complete protein.

Foods that Cause Fatigue

Some foods are especially hard to digest and thus create ama. Remember that ama is the toxic, sticky sludge that gums up your body's channels. Ama can block the channels conveying nutrient fluids to the cells (essentially starving the cells) and can block the channels of elimination, keeping the toxins in the cells instead of flowing out the body as they should. The result is that you feel sluggish, low on energy, and toxic.

One of the main foods that drain energy is red meat (including beef, pork, veal, and venison. Red meat is very heavy and difficult to digest, and thus is a major contributor of ama. Even Western physicians are beginning to note the benefits of a vegetarian diet in reducing heart disease, colon cancer, and other chronic illnesses.

Other fatigue-causing foods include mushrooms, potatoes, peanuts, fermented foods such as alcohol, vinegary foods, smoked or pickled foods, aged foods (such as cheeses), and, as mentioned earlier, any leftovers, packaged, frozen, or canned foods. Processed foods pose an additional problem: they contain many additives, chemicals and preservatives--and these tax the body's digestive system, creating extra toxins.

Most packaged foods, even breads and crackers, contain unhealthy fats such as hydrogenated vegetable oils, which are difficult for the body to digest and contribute to elevated cholesterol levels. So it's best to avoid packaged foods, and to cook your own foods with ghee or olive oil.

About Meat:

While the vegetarian diet is recommended by Maharishi Vedic Medicine because it is the most energy-giving and sattvic, as mentioned before, it's not a good idea to turn into a vegetarian overnight. You could start by having one or two purely vegetarian meals a week, and by incorporating more "white" meat into your diet (such as chicken, turkey, or fish) to replace the red meat. If you feel better, and start experiencing more energy, then you can add more vegetarian meals and less and less meat meals. In this way, you will gradually adjust to a vegetarian diet, based on the experience of more and more energy.

A Precaution:

It's important to get enough protein, especially if you are fatigued. You can do this by combining beans and grains (as all traditional cultures do), adding organic dairy products such as fresh, non-aged cheeses (cottage cheese, ricotta, and panir) and also by eating moderate amounts of tofu and other soy-based proteins.

About Genetically Engineered Foods:

Foods grown with pesticides and chemicals can be energy-drainers. These foreign, inedible toxins clog the system and stymie the digestion. That's why organic foods are so important.

There is another reason to eat organic--in recent years, many genetically modified (GMO) foods have entered our food supply. Much of the soy, corn, potatoes and tomatoes in the U.S. have been genetically altered. In many cases, the genes of these vegetables have been spliced with genes of other species--a cold-water fish gene, for instance, has been spliced with tomato genes to create a tomato that can withstand frost. In other cases, genes of bacteria, pesticides, and even viruses have been spliced with food genes to create certain effects.

Many scientists in Europe and the U.S. are concerned that these foods have not been thoroughly tested for their impact on humans, especially for people with allergies who may unwittingly eat the very food they are allergic to (you may think you're eating a tomato, but there's part fish in there). As one example, epidemiologists have noted that a dramatic rise in soy allergies has coincided with the introduction of genetically modified soy several years ago.

In general, a good rule of thumb is that food is best when it is whole, unprocessed, genetically normal, and organic. That is the most pure, sattvic, and energy-giving food--just how nature made it.

About Stimulants:

People who suffer from fatigue often resort to stimulants such as coffee, caffeinated tea, and alcohol. This is a big mistake. First of all, stimulants can mask the symptoms of fatigue and prevent you from seeking the help you need until the imbalance is farther along (and harder to treat). Secondly, caffeine and alcohol tax the liver, which is responsible for removing toxins from the body. When your liver is overloaded, toxins tend to build up, creating even greater fatigue and leading to other illnesses as well.

An abhyanga (ayurvedic oil massage), as described in Chapter Eight, is a much healthier and more enjoyable way to wake up and energize your mind and body in the morning. The massage enlivens the energy points in the body, increases blood circulation to the brain, balances Vata dosha, and relaxes the nervous system. Its effect on the body is, in other words, the opposite of the effect of caffeine.

Plus, of course, the Transcendental Meditation program, which sharpens up your thinking, energizes you and sends you out into the day with top notch clarity of mind.

About Microwave Cooking:

In recent years many people have become accustomed to "nuking" their food in a microwave. There are two reasons why this may not be so healthy for you. One is that it does not cook the food in the traditional way, by heating it gently. Instead, it changes the polarity of the water molecules in the food at about 2450 million times per second, which creates heat. It is possible that this procedure destroys the prana in food.

Secondly, when you cook with a microwave, the food does not produce any mouth-watering smells. Smelling the food is an important step in the digestive process, because when you smell bread baking, for instance, your mouth starts to water. The digestive process actually starts in your mouth when the saliva starts to break down the food, before it even enters the stomach. Smelling the food causes digestive saliva to form in the mouth, and digestive juices to form in the stomach. These enhance digestion.

You might want to try cooking a meal on the stove just to see how you feel. Are you more aware of the smell, taste, color, and texture of the food? Do you feel more satisfied, more light and happy after eating?

It's very likely.

Foods for Balancing the Doshas

Besides recommending an overall sattvic diet, Maharishi Vedic Medicine recommends certain foods to balance certain doshas. This is based on a simple classification of foods according to six tastes: sweet, sour, salty, astringent, bitter, and pungent.

Sweet foods include rice, wheat, and most breads; milk, cream, butter, ghee and other sweet dairy products; sweet fruits such as dates, cherries, and grapes; sweet vegetables such as squash, carrots, and beets.

Sour foods include yogurt, sour cream, and sour cheeses; lemons, limes, grapefruit, sour oranges, sour cherries; fermented foods such as soy sauce; foods made with vinegar such as pickles

Salty foods include any foods with high salt content, such as chips.

Bitter foods include green leafy vegetables such as spinach, chard, parsley, endive; vegetables such as cabbage, broccoli, cauliflower, brussel sprouts and spices such as turmeric.

Astringent foods include legumes such as beans, lentils, split mung beans; walnuts; honey; salad greens and sprouts; many raw vegetables; apples, persimmons, and berries.

Pungent include hot spices such as chilies, black pepper, mustard seeds, ginger, cumin, and garlic; spicy vegetables such as red radish, onions and daikon radish.

All six tastes need to be included in every meal to create a balanced diet. In fact, many imbalances can result if one of the tastes is omitted. At the same time, the six tastes can be varied in quantity to balance the doshas, and can become powerful tools for healing chronic fatigue and other illnesses. In the next section, you'll learn how.

The Qualities of Food to Balance the Doshas

There are other qualities that food can have, such as warm, cold, dry, oily, light or heavy. Soups are warm and moist; crackers are light and dry. Do you remember that discussion of your doshas in Chapter 3? Well, if you want to increase a certain dosha, you should eat foods that have similar qualities. Similar qualities increase the dosha, whereas opposite qualities decrease it.

In other words, if you want to decrease vata, you will want to eat foods that have opposite qualities to the cold, dry, moving vata-- foods that are heavy, oily, warm, sweet, sour, and salty to be exact. If you want to increase vata, you'll eat foods that are also dry, light, cold, bitter, astringent and pungent.

Let's say you have a pitta imbalance, which means that you have an excess of sharp, hot, sour qualities in your constitution. What would a meal composed of tomato soup, salty chips, Southwestern corn bread with chilies, and lemonade do to you? You guessed it--all those hot, sour, salty foods would increase your pitta.

You'd be better off eating a meal like this: cream of asparagus soup, salad, carrot muffins, and sweet lassi. These sweet, astringent and bitter tasting foods would cool the fiery pitta and create more balance in your body.

Individualized Dietary Guidelines to Balance Chronic Fatigue

As mentioned earlier, chronic fatigue is usually a vata, kapha or vata-kapha disorder. If there are other diseases present, other doshic imbalances could be involved as well.

When you consult a physician trained in Maharishi Vedic Medicine, he or she will conduct a pulse diagnosis to determine the underlying doshic imbalances. Depending on what your pulse diagnosis reveals, your physician will prescribe a diet to correct your specific imbalances. The foods prescribed will balance vata, pitta, or kapha according to the following principles. These guidelines are also used to balance the doshas during the different seasons.

To Balance Vata Dosha (or during vata Season) - Increase foods that are sweet, sour, salty, warm, nourishing. Decrease foods that are bitter, astringent, pungent, cold, dry, and light.

To Balance Pitta Dosha (or during pitta Season) - Increase foods that are sweet, bitter, astringent, cool, heavy, and oily. Decrease foods that are sour, salty, pungent, hot, light, and dry.

Kapha Pacifying Tastes (or during kapha Season) - Increase foods that are bitter, astringent, pungent, light, dry, and warm. Decrease foods that are sweet, sour, salty, heavy, oily, and cold.

A Suggested Diet for Chronic Fatigue:

The following foods balance vata and are easy to digest, and thus are often recommended for people with Chronic Fatigue. Of course, additional foods would be added or subtracted by your physician according to your doshas and health needs.

Whole grains: rice, cous cous, and whole wheat flour

Spices: turmeric, cumin, fresh ginger, black pepper, saffron, coriander leaf, coriander seed, coriander powder, black mustard seed, lemon juice for seasoning.

Dairy: warm milk with saffron; sweet buttermilk; lassi

Vegetables: okra, pumpkin, squashes, bottle gourd, cherry tomato, coriander leaf, lemon, fresh ginger,

Fruits: pomegranate, sweet oranges, sweet peaches, sweet grapes, kiwi, watermelon, sweet apples, sweet cherries, sweet tangerines.

Increase: Freshly cooked, warm foods and warm soups

Avoid: nuts; oily, deep-fried, hard-to-digest foods; very spicy foods; alcohol; onion and garlic; root vegetables such as potatoes.

CHAPTER 12

Digestion is the Key

Since I've just spent the last chapter talking about the importance of a healthy diet in combating fatigue, you may be surprised when I say that there is something even more important than diet: healthy digestion. If your digestion were strong, if the "crusher" were truly powerful, then you could digest anything. You could literally make ojas out of poison.

Digestion is such a central aspect of Maharishi Vedic Medicine that almost all treatment, for almost all diseases, starts with digestion.

What is meant by a healthy digestion? As you learned in Chapter 3, agni, the digestive fire, must be burning brightly. If agni is strong enough, it will burn away the ama in the body, and if it is balanced, it will turn food into ojas.

Diet is intertwined with this--one of the main ways to balance agni is to eat a light, easily digested diet that does not include ama-producing foods, as you've learned in this chapter.

There are also powerful purification procedures, such as Maharishi Rejuvenation Therapy, which we have discussed, which resets the agni. Maharishi Ayur-Veda herbal formulas also help.

Signs of Balanced and Imbalanced Digestion

How do you know if your digestion is going well? One way to tell is how you feel after you eat a main meal. Do you feel a light, satisfied feeling after the meal, a feeling of comfort after eating? Does the food seem to "go down" easily, and do you feel more energy from eating? Do you feel hungry before the next meal begins?

If your digestion is in trouble, you might feel gas, bloating, heartburn, dullness, lethargy, and fatigue after a meal. You might feel the need to sleep. And even after four or five hours, you may still feel stuffed, even when it's time for the next meal.

There are three main types of digestive imbalances, associated with the three doshas, vata, pitta and kapha.

Three Types of Digestive Imbalance

Vata imbalance: characterized by irregular digestion, and usually associated with gas, bloating, constipation

Pitta imbalance (tikshna): characterized by a burning sensation in the stomach,

Kapha imbalance: characterized by slow digestion, fullness and dullness after eating

How Digestive Imbalances Lead to Chronic Fatigue

A weak digestion is common as one of the primary causes of chronic fatigue. It's often at the root of other disorders that the CF patient suffers from as well. When agni is weakened, ama accumulates, and ama then becomes a major factor in creating Chronic Fatigue symptoms. It blocks the anavaha srotas, the channels that carry food and energy to the cells. The cells become tired and you become fatigued.

What causes agni to be weakened in the first place is a variety of factors, including irregular eating habits, eating before the previous meal is digested, eating too little or too much, eating a diet that is not suited for your doshas, eating a tamasic diet, or an irregular daily routine.

Once fatigue sets in, a vicious cycle gets created. This is because fatigue usually causes you to become even more irregular in your routine and eating habits. If you are very tired, you may not have the energy to cook a wholesome meal, so you may even skip meals.

Once ama creates fatigue in the body, it can also disrupt sleeping patterns and cause emotional and psychological imbalances, which in turn, affect digestion further. It becomes difficult to break this cycle when you are too tired to do anything.

With the help of a physician trained in Maharishi Vedic Medicine, you can break out of the cycle. By following the dietary suggestions (above) you can do quite a lot. Here are some concrete suggestions for improving your digestion. These are simple to do, and do not take much time or energy.

Ways to Enhance Digestion

There are some simple things you can do to boost your digestion--and eliminate fatigue. Here are ten guidelines to follow.

1. Sit down while you eat. If you eat standing up or eat on the run, digestion is interrupted and, you guessed it, ama gets formed instead of ojas.

2. Give your meal the attention it deserves. The art of eating requires that you actually taste the food--and enjoy its smell, colors, textures, and arrangement on the plate. For this reason, it's not a good idea to eat in front of the TV, to have intense discussions or arguments while eating, to talk while you have food in your mouth, or to talk on the phone. Light conversation is best. It's also a good idea to choose a quiet, settled place to eat the food rather than a crowded, noisy restaurant. By giving the food, and your digestion, your full attention, it will facilitate the smooth breakdown of food.

3. Don't overeat. Maharishi Vedic Medicine recommends that you fill your stomach with 1/3 food, 1/3 liquid, and 1/3 air. This gives a little space for the digestive process to take place in. It also prevents you from overeating and producing ama.

4. After eating, stay seated for at least two minutes before leaving the table. This extra bit of rest gives your digestion a chance to get off to the right start. If you have the time, you could even stay seated for five or ten minutes, just to allow digestion to take place smoothly. A moderately-paced ten to fifteen minute walk after the meal also helps digestion. For more intensive exercise, it's better to wait a couple of hours after the meal.

Before the meal, taking half a minute to catch your breath and to notice the food before biting into it is a good idea. Most religious traditions teach people to stop for a moment to pray over the food, to give thanks to God and to offer a blessing. This has a physiological effect of settling the mind and body before eating.

5. Don't eat in between meals. Wait for at least 2 1/2 hours after eating a full meal to begin eating again. The digestive process takes time. If you interrupt it with a new batch of food, it's kind of like introducing raw beans to a pot of beans that have been cooking for two hours. You'd end up with a half-raw, half-burned meal. In other words, ama. That's why it's so important not to snack between meals unless you're actually hungry, and won't be eating again for a few hours.

6. Eat the main meal at noon rather than evening. This is because the internal digestive fire (agni) is strongest when the sun is at its zenith in the sky (between 12:00 and 1:00 p.m.). The microcosm reflects the macrocosm. The increased digestive fire makes it easier to digest a heavy meal. Certain foods, such as meat, fried foods, tofu, cheese, and yogurt, are best eaten at noon, when the digestion is strong enough to handle them. The noon meal should also be the biggest in quantity.

If you eat a big meal with lots of heavy, difficult to digest foods at night, you will probably not be able to digest it completely before bed, and thus ama will be created. One of the most important things you can do to increase digestion is to eat lightly at night, to match the lower digestive strength available at that time.

7. Avoid ice cold food and drink. If you eat icy things, it douses the digestive fire and makes digestion sluggish or impossible. On the other hand, sipping a small amount of room temperature water or hot water with the meal helps facilitate the digestive process.

Another point about drinks--you can melt ama simply by sipping hot water throughout the day. You can keep a supply in a thermos, and take a sip every half hour or so. The hot water helps melt ama and flushes out impurities. It also helps balance Vata dosha, which is often a major player in fatigue. This is an inexpensive way yet effective way to cleanse the digestion and increase energy.

Finally, it's important not to drink too much at a meal. Too much liquid will douse the digestive fire. Sipping a half a cup of water with the meal is usually enough liquid, especially if you are eating soup too.

8. Eat at the same time every day. The body loves regularity. If you eat breakfast, lunch and dinner at the same time every day, your digestion will become attuned to these natural cycles and will prepare itself. You'll naturally start feeling hungry right before a meal, and will be able to digest it more efficiently. Eating at regular times also balances Vata dosha, which tends to be unstable and variable by nature. Following a regular daily routine will help digestion.

9. Don't eat too fast or too slowly. Eating too fast causes you to

swallow air and disrupts the digestive process. Also, it's impossible to taste or chew the food properly if you're wolfing it down. So take time to savor it. Strangely enough, eating too slowly can also be a problem, as in a large multi-course meal that extends for more than an hour. The food eaten at the beginning of the meal will already be digesting before you get to the end! This will only amount to indigestion, ama, and low energy and dullness afterwards.

10. Taking a short, 15-minute hour walk after lunch and dinner can help stimulate digestion. Walk at a comfortable speed, without straining. By improving digestion, this can help a lot in eliminating fatigue.

11. Avoid heavy, cold and frozen, leftover, processed foods. Follow the diet that your physician trained in Maharishi Vedic Medicine gives you to balance your doshas and create a balanced digestion.

Balanced Elimination

Elimination is the other half of digestion. Constipation is often a vata (drying) disorder, and is also affected by lack of exercise, eating tamasic foods, eating irregularly, sleep problems, not drinking enough water during the day, and sleeping during the day.

If your body is not eliminating waste properly, toxins and ama can build up. Constipation is the result of weak digestion, and when it manifests, it can weaken digestion even further. If left untreated, constipation can eventually result in disease.

Some of the suggestions a physician trained in Maharishi Vedic Medicine might recommend are: drink more warm water throughout the day; eating Vata-pacifying foods; following the Ayurvedic daily routine, with regular times for eating, sleeping and activity; eating more sweet oranges, cooked pears, and cooked prunes; soaking a 1/2 cup of raisins in a cup of water during the day and eating them before bed, chewing carefully; eating psyllium seed husk, soaked overnight in room temperature water, add honey and eat like cereal; taking an early-morning walk or walking briefly after meals; drinking a cup of warm milk with ghee before bed; and taking prescribed herbal formulas to stimulate regular bowel movements.

Remember that ama blocks the flow of energy in the body. In this chapter you've learned to avoid the factors that create indigestion, such as irregular meals, eating too fast or slow, drinking too much fluid, cold/frozen foods, eating between meals, leftover foods, very oily food, overly spicy food, meat products, root vegetables and beans, and heavy foods.

Following these simple suggestions will help you to reduce ama and create ojas--and will help boost your energy levels considerably.

CHAPTER 13

Energizing the Environment

I have not yet talked about the role of environmental factors in creating Chronic Fatigue. Diseases such as "sick building syndrome" have been highly publicized in recent years. The use of toxic materials in carpeting, paints, insulation, and glues have led to thousands of employees getting sick. Fatigue is one of the main symptoms, along with headaches, congestion, dizziness, nausea, sore throat, skin irritation, rash, wheezing, difficulty breathing, and tightness in the chest.

Recent research at Cornell University suggests that it's not the toxins from building materials so much as a build-up in carbon dioxide caused by a lack of fresh air. The researchers point out that sick building syndrome surfaced in the 1980s, when energy-conscious architects designed buildings to be air-tight. Other causes might be the lighting, the chairs, and air pollutants.

Whatever the exact cause, the fact is that buildings and furnishings are designed in such a way that people are getting sick. In this situation, the most a worker could hope for is that the irritating factors, such as lack of fresh air or pollutants, could be removed from the workplace.

But what if a building or a home could be designed to actually make a person's health better? If certain buildings could make you sick, then couldn't some be designed to make you feel more energy, better health?

One of the approaches of Maharishi Vedic Medicine does exactly that. In the sophisticated science of building design called Sthapatya Veda,[28] everything about the home or workplace is designed to create mental, physical, emotional, social, and even financial health.

The word "Sthapatya" is derived from the Sanskrit root "stha," meaning "established." The idea of Sthapatya Veda is to create buildings that enable their occupants to become established in natural law, to live in harmony with the laws of nature that govern the universe and our own bodies.

Many people today do not realize that the buildings that they live and work in could be making them sick and causing other serious problems. Ill-health, loss of money, and other misfortunes can result when the building is designed in ways that are not in harmony with nature. Anxiety, depression, illness, chronic disease, blocks to creativity, bad luck, financial loss, obstacles to progress and success, disharmony in relationships and the breakdown of the family are all results of poorly designed buildings.

On the other hand, people who live in buildings that are designed in harmony with Natural Law report a variety of positive results. These include more energy and less fatigue, more alertness and vitality throughout the day, more restful and refreshing sleep, more clear and creative thinking, better decision-making, greater health and

28. http://www.sthapatyaveda.com/

happiness, greater peace of mind and less stress.

Just as disease is caused by a violation of laws of nature, a building can cause disease in its occupants if it is not built in harmony with nature.

How do you go about building a home or office in accord with Natural Law? The Vedic texts outline three important things to consider: direction, placement and proportion.

Direction

The sun is the greatest natural force in our universe, causing the cycles of the and the daily circadian cycles of day and night. The modern science of chronobiology measures the effect of the circadian rhythms in the body, and how the metabolism changes as the sun moves through the sky from morning to night to morning again. You have already seen how these daily and seasonal cycles play an important role in determining healthy daily and seasonal routines in Maharishi Vedic Medicine.

These cycles of the sun play an important role in building design as well. According to the Vedic texts, every building needs to face the right direction in order to make maximum use of the sun's energy as it moves across the sky. The most auspicious direction is east, because the sun's energy is vital and fresh in the morning when it rises. If the entrance to the building faces east, then the revitalizing, positive energy of the sun enters the building and brings health and vitality to the family living in it.

There are inauspicious directions as well, and the most inauspicious of these is south. If the entrance to the building faces south, it can bring ill health, lack of energy, loss of wealth, and misfortune to the occupants. Other inauspicious directions for the entrance to face are northeast, northwest, southeast, southwest, and, to a lesser degree, west.

Besides east, north is the only other auspicious direction for the entrance of the home or office building. This means that seventy-five percent of homes and offices are currently facing an inauspicious direction, and are bringing unhealthy influences to the people living or working there.

There may be a physiological reason for this. Research shows that certain neurons in the brain fire differently depending on the direction the person is facing. That may be the reason why the Vedic texts recommend facing east for important activities such as cooking, studying, working, and meditating. In a Sthapatya Veda home, the stove, desks, and meditation chairs will all face east.

Placement

As the sun moves across the sky, it strikes different areas of your home, creating different energy levels throughout the day. The Vedic texts describe the precise placement of various rooms in the house to make the maximum use of this revitalizing energy.

The kitchen, for instance, is placed in the southeast corner of the home, where the sun's energy is greatest at noon, when the main meal is cooked. This energizes the cooking of the food, and in fact, the best placement of the stove is in the southwest corner of the kitchen.

The living room is placed in the west, because people usually occupy it in the later part of the day, when the sun's energy still lingers, and there is a relaxing, settled energy created by the sun at that time. Every room is placed in the spot where the quality of the sun will enhance the activity that is usually conducted in that room.

Modern architects, who have no inkling of the power and influence of the sun, unwittingly place rooms in the wrong areas of the house, bringing ill health to the occupants. The Vedic texts actually mention chronic fatigue as a result of wrong placement of rooms, and specify which placements can cause other health problems. For instance, the wrong placement of the kitchen brings digestive imbalances, and the wrong placement of the bedroom can cause insomnia or chronic fatigue.

In the Vedic home, there is an ideal place for relaxing, bathing, cooking, eating, sleeping, and studying or working.

There is another level to this analysis in addition to the solar component, in that each of the directions is considered to embody or have a quality of one or more of the elements such as space (east), fire (southeast), water (northeast), earth (southwest). These principles also affect room placement in that the southwest corner would be considered a more grounded place that is compatible with sleep, the southeast a better place for the cooking process, and the northeast a better place for alert yet quiet meditation.

Proportion

Throughout the ages, the perfect proportions of the human body have fascinated artists. Leonardo da Vinci, who studied anatomy in order to learn how to draw the human body, revealed that the body is a perfect expression of nature's balance.

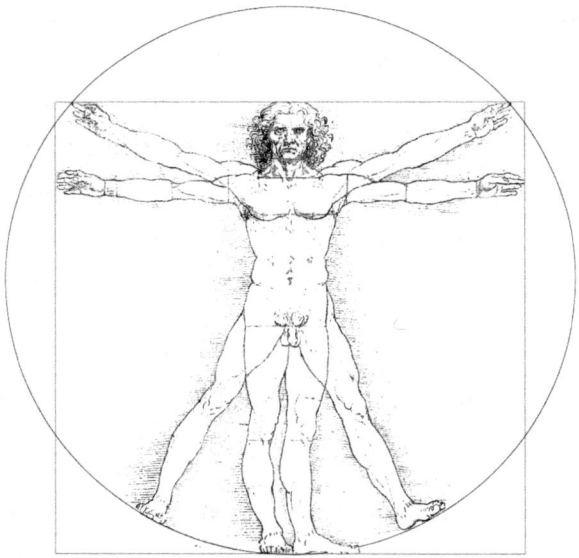

Proportion is found throughout nature. The "golden mean" is a balanced design that ancient mathematicians discovered existing in nature, imbedded in the perfect spiral of a conch shell and the proportion of petals unfolding in a flower blossom.

The idea is that the home you live in should reflect these perfect proportions of the human body and of nature as a whole. When the dimensions of each room are designed in proportion to every other room and to the building as a whole, then harmony and a sense of balance is created in the awareness of the people living or working there.

Ideal Vastu

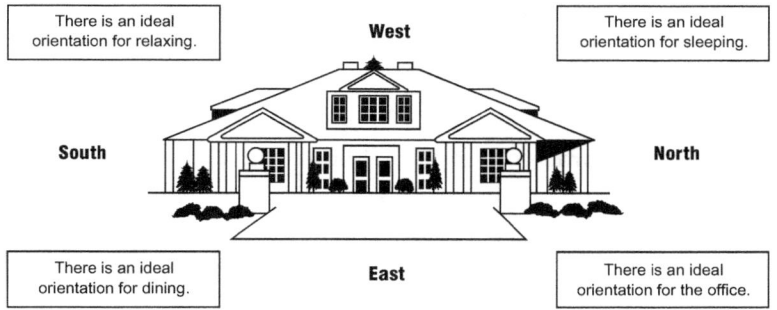

"Vastu," is another important concept in Maharishi Sthapatya Veda. "Vastu" is a Sanskrit word meaning "holistic structure of Natural Law," and it refers to the relationship between a building, its site, and the near and far environment. It establishes a connection between the individual and the sun, moon, stars, and universe.

Vastu can be auspicious or inauspicious, depending on its orientation, shape, and placement in reference to bodies of water, slope of land, and other geographical factors. An auspicious vastu is square or rectangular in shape, precisely aligned with the four directions. The boundaries of the vastu would face squarely north, south, east, and west, with the entrance to the vastu on the east. A low wall or fence defines the boundaries of the vastu, and it is placed on the property so that any slopes fall to the north or east. The home or office building is placed inside the vastu, and, as mentioned earlier, it should also face true east.

Brahmasthan

When people enter a building designed with the principles of Maharishi Sthapatya Ved, they often comment on how silent it feels. This silence effect is largely due to an interesting design element called a Brahmasthan. The Brahmasthan is an empty space in the center of the home or office building which provides a core of silence and pure consciousness. All of the other rooms are placed around the Brahmasthan, just as all of the activity in the mind takes place on the basis of pure consciousness.

"I feel there is a silence you can almost touch and hear. . .it's really solid, a feeling of completeness," comments David Perez, a resident in the Rukmapura Park hotel in Fairfield, Iowa, a Maharishi Sthapatya Veda designed building. Other residents, Dr. Lee Fergusson and Dr. Anna Bonshek comment, "We seem affected by the way the light enters the building. Every day as we rise and go about our daily activity, it is as if the sun is following our every move, supporting us every step of the way. We experience a tangible sense of connectedness with the movement of the sun, and through it, a more profound feeling of integration with the cosmos."

Designing Healthy Communities

The science of Maharishi Sthapatya Ved does not stop with the healthy design of single buildings. Entire communities can be designed according to these principles, with the roads, utilities, public buildings, parks, and individual homes all designed to bring health and vitality to the individuals living there. The roads, for instance, should be on an east-west axis in order to bring sufficient air flow into the community.

At the heart of the community is a brahmasthan, to create a silent, coherent core of nourishing qualities for the entire community. In the home the brahmasthan is an empty space; in the community it's a large park or garden for everyone to enjoy. And around the edges of the community, the Vedic texts recommend planting a wide buffer zone of forest, in order to provide adequate oxygen and green space for the community to thrive in a stress-free environment.

Other features that are included in designing ideal communities are site planning, layout with each house oriented to the east, low-density housing, nontoxic and energy-efficient construction, adequate fresh air, generous green space, nonpolluting vehicles, and sustainable organic agricultural areas to grow healthy food for the entire community.

Effects of the Distant Environment on Chronic Fatigue

If you suffer from Chronic Fatigue or Chronic Fatigue Syndrome, you probably have spent a good amount of time wondering "why me?" The symptoms of CF and CFS can be so debilitating, so completely devastating, that all normal life screeches to a halt. Yet because the doctors often cannot locate organic causes for CF or CFS, chronic fatigue sufferers sometimes have a tough time explaining their illness to others. Fortunately, the condition is now much more recognized by the medical community and the public, thanks to more increased public awareness in the past fifteen years, but still the question remains, "Why me?" The disease can hit so suddenly. One day you're running a business, raising a family, and getting a graduate degree, and the next day you suddenly find that you can't get out of bed.

One explanation lies in the field of Maharishi Jyotish, or Vedic astrology, which is one of the 40 aspects of Maharishi Vedic Medicine. Maharishi Jyotish explains how different influences from the distant environment--the influence of the sun, moon, stars, planetscan affect your health.

So far you've been hearing about ways that the near environment can provide energy, good health and life-giving qualities if it is properly designed. That is already a fairly unusual concept. But Maharishi Vedic Medicine doesn't stop there. It takes into account the far environmentthe influence of the cosmos on your healthas well.

Maharishi Vedic Astrology calculates the cycles of time that bring about transformations in your life. This is possible because according to Maharishi Vedic Science, life unfolds sequentially in predictable cycles, based on predictable laws of nature. From this perspective, all of nature, from the tiniest amoeba to the far distant galaxies, is governed by the same laws of nature.

Think of an automobile production line. If you know the sequence of steps involved in producing a car, you can look at that car at any one point in its development and know which steps have been completed and which remain. Similarly, the Maharishi Vedic Astrology consultation looks at one point in a person's life, the birth time, and uses that point to predict trends and cycles in the future.

With Maharishi Vedic Astrology, you can find out future trends in your health, career, finances, relationships and family life. It's like creating a map of your future, with all the ups and downs laid out before you. This is extremely useful in preventing ill health, because Maharishi Vedic Medicine also offers ways to transform negative trends into positive ones.

One of the main principles of Maharishi Vedic Medicine is "avert the danger before it arises" (heyam dukham anagatam). This is the key idea of Maharishi Vedic Astrology.

It's also useful if you are already in a negative cycle, for instance, if you are already suffering from Chronic Fatigue or Chronic Fatigue Syndrome. Maharishi Vedic Astrology can tell you how long the current state will last, what factors are causing the problem, and will give you solutions to remedy the situation.

Let's look at the four major elements of this ancient science of prediction, so you can understand how it can help you in your fight against Chronic Fatigue.

Nine Grahas (Planets)

You could think of the grahas, or planets, as administrators in the universe. For instance, Surya (the sun) represents pure consciousness; Chandra (the moon) represents the cosmic mind, and Budha (Mercury) represents the cosmic intellect. Because individual life is governed by the same laws of nature that govern the whole universe, these grahas govern similar areas in your own life, with Budha (Mercury) ruling the intellect, and Chandra (the moon) ruling the mind and emotions. Together, the nine grahas govern all aspects of individual and cosmic life.

The following list includes the nine grahas, with their Sanskrit and English names, and their abbreviations. The first seven are visible in the sky; the last two are points in space where the moon's path appears to intersect with the sun's path.

The Nine Grahas (Planets)		
Abbreviation	**Sanskrit Name**	**English Name**
Sy	Surya	Sun
Ch	Chandra	Moon
Ma	Mangala	Mars
Bu	Budha	Mercury
Gu	Guru	Jupiter
Sk	Shukra	Venus
Sa	Shani	Saturn
Rh	Rahu	Ascending lunar node*
Kt	Ketu	Descending lunar node*

Maharishi Vedic Astrology pinpoints the exact time and nature of the influences of these grahas on your life. This allows you to prevent future bouts of ill health or misfortune, and helps you to eliminate negative influences that are active right now, or about to become active.

The Twelve Rashis (Signs of the Zodiac)

The Vedic texts conceptualize the universal body as having the same form as the human body. The body of the universe consists of twelve rashis, which you may recognize as astrological signs of the zodiac. Each rashi represents a different part of the body of the universe, and different part of your body.

The grahas move through the twelve signs, creating effects in different rashis. If a graha brings a negative effect to the first rashi, it could result in a negative effect on your head or your overall health. Other rashis correspond to the eyes, the neck and shoulders, the chest, and so on.

The sun moves through the twelve rashis in the solar cycle of a year, while the moon moves through in the lunar cycle of twenty-eight days. Other grahas take varying amounts of time, depending on their speed of movement.

Here are the twelve rashis with their Sanskrit and English names.

The Twelve Rashis (Constellations)		
Number	Sanskrit Name	English Name
1	Mesha	Aries
2	Vrishabha	Taurus
3	Mithuna	Gemini
4	Karka	Cancer
5	Sinha	Leo
6	Kanya	Virgo
7	Tula	Libra
8	Vrishchika	Scorpio
9	Dhanu	Sagittarius
10	Makara	Capricorn
11	Kumbha	Aquarius
12	Meena	Pisces

* The two lunar nodes are the points in space where the moon's path appears to intersect the sun's path, as viewed from the Earth.

The Twenty-Seven Nakshatras

A nakshatra is a cluster of stars within each rashi, or sign of the zodiac. Each rashi is composed of two or more nakshatras. The Sanskrit word nakshatra means "that which does not decay." The twenty-seven nakshatras represent the imperishable nature of consciousness itself, which never grows old or changes.

The nakshatras, like consciousness, permeate the universe. They create specific qualities within the rashi they are positioned in, and also influence the grahas. In other words, a graha will take on a different quality depending on the nakshatra it is positioned in, and thus will create different effects in your life.

The moon passes through the cycle of twenty-seven nakshatras in the course of 28 days. Thus it takes slightly more than a day to pass through each one.

Interpreting the Janma Kundali, or Birth Chart

The planets (grahas) move through the rashis and nakshatras at their own speed. The Janma Kundali, or birth chart, is like a snapshot of the position of the grahas at the exact time of your birth. To cast a birth chart, your date, time and geographical location at birth are used.

The grahas at the time of your birth were in a specific position, occupying different rashis and nakshatras. Each graha is positioned in specific rashi and different nakshatra, which governs a particular aspect of the body.

There is also a consideration of the placement of grahas in particular bhavas, or "houses" in your particular chart. Bhava placement governs different areas of life, such as health, wealth, home, education, partnership and marriage, education, good fortune, spiritual life, and career.

The birth chart provides a blueprint for the probable direction of your life, from which predictions can be made for your future.

Here is an example of a birth chart, which is divided into twelve squares to represent the rashis and bhavas. The planets are represented by their abbreviations, the rashis, represented by their numbers, are placed according to the rashi that is rising on the horizon at the time of birth. The bhavas always follow the same pattern, with the first one starting in the upper middle square.

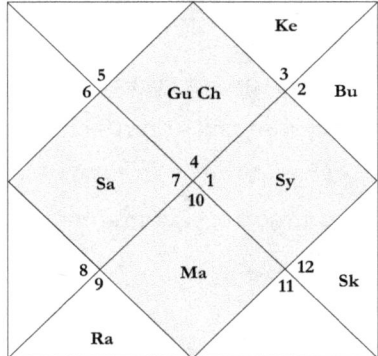

There are other influences that must be taken into account, such as the position of the planets in the sky right now. At a consultation with a Maharishi Vedic Pundit, you can find out what the primary trends are in your life, what's happening right now, and what the trends and events will be like in the future.

Discovering the Root Cause of Chronic Fatigue

As mentioned earlier in this book, it is often difficult for the physician to discover the underlying cause of Chronic Fatigue and CFS, because they involve multiple disorders and layers of imbalance. One of the practical uses of the Maharishi Jyotish program is to locate which grahas have created the illness. Maharishi Jyotish pandits (Vedic experts) are able to identify those influences, and can then recommend remedial measures to help remove those negative influences being created by the grahas. This can greatly support the other medical treatments for Chronic Fatigue.

Changing the Trends of Time

Let's say that you have a Maharishi Jyotish consultation and found out that you are in a period of ill-health that will last for another three years. You are disappointed to find out that you won't be well right away, but you're relieved to hear that at least you don't have to suffer the rest of your life. What you really want to know is, what can I do to relieve my situation right now?

As part of your consultation, the pandit will prescribe specific performances, called the Maharishi Yagyas, to change the negative influence into a positive one. These performances, which have been enlivened in recent times by Maharishi Mahesh Yogi, are described in Vedic texts in many places, and were a vital feature of the ancient Vedic civilization, which enjoyed peace, prosperity, and good health for many thousands of years.

They are conducted by Vedic pandits, trained in India under Maharishi's guidance, to perform the yagyas on the basis of their own experience of the silent level of pure consciousness. It is this proper training that creates such good results.

The Maharishi Yagya Program creates life-supporting influences to remove unwanted tendencies before they happen. If there is a problem in ill health, finances, or relationships seen in the future, the Maharishi Yagya Program can help avert the danger before it happens.

The performances work on the principle of action and reaction. All of our thoughts, words and actions create influences in our environment, and these influences come back to us. If you've ever thrown a stone into a small pond, you know how this works. The stone makes a splash and then sends a series of concentric ripples that keep expanding until they reach the edges of the pond--and then they start rippling back until they reach the point where the stone first entered the water and created the first ripple.

With your birth chart, the Maharishi Vedic Pandit is able to analyze the influences that have been created by your past actions, and can predict the exact time that these influences will come to you. If the influence is not positive, then a Maharishi Yagya performance will be prescribed to create the exact life-supporting influence that you need to neutralize the negativity coming to you. And if the influence coming to you is positive, a Maharishi Yagya can enhance that positive influence.

Creating Balance Between Individual and Cosmic Life

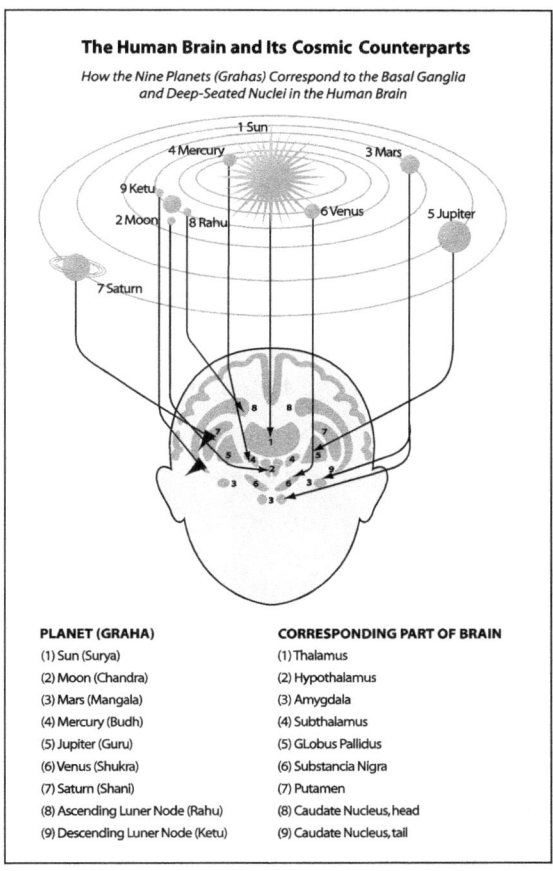

The Human Brain and Its Cosmic Counterparts

How the Nine Planets (Grahas) Correspond to the Basal Ganglia and Deep-Seated Nuclei in the Human Brain

PLANET (GRAHA)	CORRESPONDING PART OF BRAIN
(1) Sun (Surya)	(1) Thalamus
(2) Moon (Chandra)	(2) Hypothalamus
(3) Mars (Mangala)	(3) Amygdala
(4) Mercury (Budh)	(4) Subthalamus
(5) Jupiter (Guru)	(5) GLobus Pallidus
(6) Venus (Shukra)	(6) Substancia Nigra
(7) Saturn (Shani)	(7) Putamen
(8) Ascending Luner Node (Rahu)	(8) Caudate Nucleus, head
(9) Descending Luner Node (Ketu)	(9) Caudate Nucleus, tail

Just like the old saying, "an ounce of prevention is worth a pound of cure," the Maharishi Yagya program is most effective when it is used to prevent problems before they happen rather than trying to stop them midstream. However, they still provide a powerful wave of relief to people who are already suffering from ill health or other problems.

Remember that perfect health is a state of balance, and balance means not just within the mind and body, but between the individual and the universe. By removing the negative influences, a level of harmony is created between the different aspects of the body, between the cosmic body and its counterparts in your own body.

This existence of "cosmic counterparts" was first introduced by Tony Nader, M.D., Ph.D., who discovered a precise one-to-one relationship between the fundamental structures and functions of the human physiology and the fundamental structures of Natural Law. For instance, Surya, the sun, which exists in the cosmos, is directly correlated with the functions of the thalamus in the human body. The following diagram shows this correlation.

The Science of Sound

The Maharishi Yagya program uses the science of sound to create the effects of balance in the individual and the environment. In fact, all of the approaches of Maharishi Vedic Medicine use sound to create balance and harmony. This is because sound is the finest level of expression in the Veda. The sounds of the Veda unfold in a fixed sequence of syllables alternated with gaps of silence. These primordial sounds are the first manifestation of consciousness, the Veda, and all matter and even the human body is composed of sound.

While the primordial nature of sound has been understood for thousands of years by Vedic experts, quantum physics has caught up to this reality in the last century. One of the groundbreaking discoveries was that particles of matter also have a wave motion, a sound or vibrational quality.

Consider that, from this perspective, the body is made of the sounds of the Veda. This is an amazing concept. It has enormous implications for healing. The sounds of the Veda can be used to evoke the memory of wholeness in the body. Sound can also be used to repair specific imbalances, because by using the correct vibration, or sound, to enliven the memory of correct functioning in a specific part of the body.

This is the principle behind all of the therapies of Maharishi Vedic Medicine. Even the Vedic herbal food supplements use the science of sound. This is because each herb has a specific vibrational frequency. Each part of the body has a corresponding frequency to a specific herb. The herb, then, acts like a tuning fork, helping to reset an imbalanced area in the mind or body to its natural frequency.

The prescribed herbal formula has a specific vibratory frequency, and that resonates with the part of the body that is imbalanced, restoring the memory of its proper vibrational pattern.

This is the way that herbs can target specific areas of the body-- through their vibrational qualities. They don't target the disease, but rather restore the memory of wholeness to the part of the body where that memory has broken down. Once the memory is restored in the area of imbalance, the body's own self-repair mechanisms take over, and the body heals itself. The herbs restore the memory of wholeness, as part of the healing process

Maharishi Vedic Sound Therapy

Listening to recitations of the Vedic literature being chanted by traditional pandits can actually normalize the wave function in specific parts of the body, and can create a powerful wave of coherence for the whole body. The memory of wholeness is restored through the primordial sounds of the Veda.

Maharishi Vedic Sound therapy helps to restore the memory of wholeness by using the primordial sounds of the Veda. Like a flooded river that clears away stagnant water as it surges down a mountain, so the flood of coherence created by the sounds of the Veda clears away blocks to the memory of wholeness, restoring the original perfect design of the body.

The traditional recitations have long been known to create a harmonizing, rejuvenating, and balancing effect in the body. Now recent research has shown that this therapy has a dramatic effect on reducing the growth of cancer cells. Dr. Hari Sharma and other researchers at the Ohio State University College of Medicine found that the sounds of Sama Veda reduced the growth of human cancer cells in vitro, while the sounds of hard rock music increased growth of cancer cells.

Dr. Sharma postulated that it is the long, slow, low-pitched rhythms of Sama Veda that strengthened the low-frequency vibrations of normal DNA, at the same time inhibiting the growth of the high-frequency vibrations of cancer cells. It will be interesting to see what further research reveals, but it is clear that these primordial sounds have a profound and orderly influence in restoring health and wholeness to the body.

Maharishi Gandharva Veda

Another type of music therapy is Maharishi Gandharva Veda. The melodies and rhythms of this classical Indian music are designed to be played at different times during the day, as the energy of the sun surges and ebbs. These cycles change every two hours, creating twelve different cycles throughout the day.

Different ragas, or musical compositions, are played during these periods to enliven the laws of nature that are lively during that time of the day. There is a distinctive flavor to night ragas as opposed to day ragas, with the night ragas being more settling and day ragas more energizing.

You could say that Gandharva Veda is the music of nature, because it enlivens the impulses of nature throughout the day and night. Nature swings in the waves of bliss, and this is the effect of Maharishi Gandharva Veda music.

By playing Maharishi Gandharva music in your home throughout the day, you can strengthen your connection to the frequencies of nature, creating more harmony, bliss, and energy. One of the effects of Maharishi Gandharva music is to create a harmonizing, peaceful influence in your home, and to neutralize stress. These are important healing influences that can make your home more restful, and a truly rejuvenating place to recover from the fatigue and stress of the workplace.

CHAPTER 14

Chronic Disease Programs

Some people don't need a memory-jogger to get back to health, they need a wake-up call. The chronic disease programs are just that, a clear bell ringing to get you up out of your illness and into the light of day. The only thing is that they'll be ringing your bell for days or even weeks at a time. Some people take a while to wake up. Oddly, with chronic fatigue, what you really want is to rest better, but, we'll get you there.

The Chronic Disease program was founded to give people with chronic illnesses in-depth treatment in the programs of Maharishi Vedic Medicine. The Maharishi Rejuvenation Centers can answer your questions about this program. [29]

Any disease that last more than two weeks or reoccurs seasonally on periodically can be considered a chronic illness. Check out the following list of illnesses addressed by the chronic disease program, and see if there is anything that anything that applies to you or someone you care about:

— Benign prostatic hyperplasia
— Bronchial asthma
— Chronic anxiety
— Chronic back pain
— Chronic bronchitis
— Chronic fatigue

— Chronic headache
— Chronic kidney disease
— Chronic liver disease
— Chronic sinusitis
— Connective tissue diseases
— Coronary heart disease

29. www.theraj.com, www.lancasterhealth.com

- Benign prostatic hyperplasia
- Bronchial asthma
- Chronic anxiety
- Chronic back pain
- Chronic bronchitis
- Chronic fatigue
- Chronic headache
- Chronic kidney disease
- Chronic liver disease
- Chronic sinusitis
- Connective tissue diseases
- Coronary heart disease
- Depression
- Diabetes
- Eczema
- Gallstones
- Hyperacidity
- Hypertension
- Hyperthyroidism
- Hypothyroidism
- Inflammatory bowel disease
- Insomnia

The people at the Maharishi Rejuvenation centers are happy to speak to you for any number of reasons, but you might be most interested in their treatment of chronic fatigue.

The program is offered under the direction of specially trained personnel. Participation begins with completion of a health-status questionnaire, which is evaluated by a staff physician in consultation with a panel of experts. The next step is personal evaluation of the patient, following which the medical staff designs an individualized program of treatment.

The usual length of the Chronic Disorders Program is 7, 14, or 21 days. During this period, patients participate in a full-time program of daily treatment as well as comprehensive health education-- instruction in how to maintain a healthy, balanced life through a system of continuing self-care. In addition to the treatment program, deluxe accommodations are provided, with gourmet organic vegetarian meals that support the prescribed regimen of therapy.

Individuals who enter the program are never asked to discontinue care provided by their family physician or specialists. The program of treatment at is closely supervised by our experienced medical staff, and may be integrated with the individual's current medications and other conventional treatments.

The Chronic Disorders program utilizes a holistic approach to enliven the body's innate healing mechanisms. This approach promotes balance by using many different modalities simultaneously. This multi-modality approach has been found to be more effective in promoting health than using single approaches individually. The program includes:

- Techniques for managing health from its foundation the field of consciousness and for alleviating the stress that frequently suppresses the body's internal self-repair mechanisms. These techniques include the Transcendental Meditation Program and TM-Sidhi program.

- A unique system of pulse diagnosis that helps the physician identify the root causes and degree of imbalance.

- Individualized Vedic purification therapies to eliminate impurities in the body that accumulate over time from improper diet, stress and other factors; such toxins or impurities may be instrumental in causing many chronic disorders.

- Rejuvenation therapy using customized herbal oil to energise each and every cell in your body.

- Maharishi Vedic Vibration Technology and Vedic Sound Therapy, technologies that utilize specific vibrations and impulses of sound to stimulate self-repair mechanisms in the body.

- Specialized herbal food supplements, traditional formulas consisting of herbs found only in certain parts of the world, to help nourish and restore balance in the body.

- Personalized program of healthy diet, individualized according to the person's constitution and pattern of underlying imbalances.

- Special exercise program tailored to the individual, including instruction in yoga exercises, balanced breathing exercises, as well as conventional exercise.

- Instruction in health-promoting behavior, including daily and seasonal routines to maintain harmony between the individual and the environment.

- Program to optimize the influence of the near environment promotion of mental and physical balance through the beneficial orientation and layout of one's home and workplace.

- Program to optimize the influence of the distant environment techniques to promote integration of the individual with the cycles and rhythms of nature, including those of the sun, moon, planets, and stars.

Most of those items should be recognizable to you on the basis of having read this book. The Maharishi Vedic Vibration Technology and Vedic Sound Therapy is described in the next chapter, so that's new.

It might be of interest to you to review scientific research on the effectiveness of these programs,[30] which, although they are new in terms of their availability in the U.S., are the world's most time-tested natural system for addressing the root cause of chronic disease.

"Root cause" is the important word here. Anyone can put a band-aid on your scraped knee. An over the counter the drug can be used to treat insomnia. Prozac can be used to treat depression. Any doctor can treat your symptoms. But this is not about that.

This is about rooting out the foundation of your illness so it has no ground on which to survive. This is about moving beyond simple recovery from illness, and moving into the prevention of illness. This is about moving past mere prevention into optimization or "super-normalization" of physiological and psychological functioning, on new levels of consciousness.

---

30. http://www.mapi.com/maharishi_ayurveda/research/index.html

We say super-normalization to distinguish it from merely average, but an enlightened state of perfect health is more truly normal, the actual birthright of every human being. It is only "super" in comparison to what most people are currently experiencing. But from the perspective of what we deserve and of what we very naturally can have, it's actually a more normal state.

It's not enough, therefore, to simply get well. Of course, many of the chronically fatigued would settle for even half well. But we have to be constantly growing in health, intelligence, and enhancing our connection with the field of pure consciousness within in order to counteract the wearing forces of stress, a challenging environment, and the passage of time. With that evolutionary process of the development of consciousness in full force, it's hard for illness and even the full force of aging to slow us down.

The Chronic Disease programs give the chronically ill the focused attention that they need to fight their illnesses, with some big weapons. So, if you are seriously ill, and if you have anything "chronic," you qualify, and you might want to look at checking yourself in for some real treatment that has a strong chance to bring you back to normal, or even way better than normal.

CHAPTER 15

About the Maharishi Vedic Vibration Therapy Program

We have talked at some length about enlivening "memory" as a means of understanding the various treatments of Maharishi Vedic Medicine. We have also looked at a model of the human physiology that looks at all creation, and certainly the human body, as wave functions or fluctuations in a larger, unified field of consciousness. From that perspective, your body can be seen as a sophisticated form of sound, an actual symphony of wave like impulses in a silent ocean of consciousness.

You've heard the sound of an orchestra warming up: a cacophony of sound, oboes bleating, violins mewing, basses plucking along, but no coordination or beauty. But then, a few taps on the conductor's stand, and the piano sounds a note. At that point everyone can attune themselves to one sound, making sure that they have the same version of the fundamental chord. Having done so, they can plunge together into a beautiful, lively aria.

There is an instantaneous galvanizing and organizing effect of that one sound. There is a similar, instantaneous effect in the programs known as the Maharishi Vedic Vibration technology.

For thousands of years, Veda and the Vedic Literature have been held to be the expression of the Total Knowledge of Natural Law, the expression of the inner intelligence of Nature which maintains and evolves human life and the life of the universe.

According to tradition, the Vedic sounds contained in Veda and the Vedic Literature are the fundamental vibrations which structure the material universe, including the human body.

We've been talking about gaining an inner attunement to these fundamental values for some time now.

Now Maharishi Vedic Vibration Experts have been trained, under Maharishi's guidance, in the proper administration of these fundamental sounds to enliven the body's inner intelligence. These sounds attune the physiology, so that, for example, through a tender impulse of Vedic vibration, pain can be transformed into a feeling of pleasantness, and abnormality can be transformed into normal physiological functioning.

This ancient understanding has recently been scientifically validated by neuroscientist Professor Tony Nader, M.D., Ph.D., who discovered an exact correlation between the structure of these Vedic vibrations and the structure and function of the human physiology. This discovery provides the rationale for correcting disorders from the most fundamental level of physiological functioning, the body's own inner intelligence.

It is remarkable to note how quickly and effortlessly Maharishi Vedic Vibration Technology can transform a state of physiological disorder into a state of orderly physiological functioning. The scientific explanation of such a sudden transformation can be derived from recent findings of the theories of Self-Organization and of Chaos Theory.

I think that you can probably relate to chaos, anyway. If you've been tired for a long time, things may not be as orderly as they used to be. It's odd to think that there is a science of chaos, but there is. Mathematical formulas have been identified to predict degrees of chaos, which seems almost contradictory: predictable chaos.

Even so, these theories of modern physics and mathematics, developed in the last few decades, have led to important scientific insights regarding the functioning of dynamic self-organizing systemsincluding the functioning of our physiology. One of the most important findings of these theories is the principle that a tender impulse can transform chaos, or disorder, into order.

Maharishi Vedic Vibration Technology utilizes this principle, and through a tender impulse of Vedic vibration, pain is transformed into a feeling of pleasantness; abnormality is transformed into normal physiological functioning; the inner intelligence of the body is enlivened in order to revitalize its physiological expression.

This is the basic principle.

This therapeutic modality is sometimes referred to as the "instant relief" program. For many people, relief is instantaneous, and only one session is enough to completely erase their symptoms. Most people have partial relief, and some need several sessions to feel full effects.

We're probably not going to instantly knock out your CFS with Maharishi Vedic Vibration Therapy, but we may be able to relieve it to some degree, at least on the symptomatic level. It may modify your CFS directly, but even some symptomatic relief may be of help. Consider for example, the following results with sleep disorders, a common corollary of chronic fatigue.

In 33 people seeking relief from sleep problems, nearly two thirds reported relief at a level of 25 percent or greater, and one third reported improvement of 50 percent or more. These figures are based on reports from participants about two weeks after their MVVT consultation. This success rate is similar to that seen in a number of other conditions. Improvements in a variety of patterns of sleep disturbance were reported. These included less difficulty in falling asleep, fewer awakenings in the night, better quality of sleep, getting adequate sleep, reduction of excess sleep, and fewer disturbing dreams.

Some of the reports were quite striking. One man had experienced sleep problems for 27 years. Although it normally took him one to two hours to fall asleep, on the night of his first session he fell asleep within 5 minutes. From then on, he had no problem falling asleep and felt fresher during the day. Three months after the consultation he reported that the relief had been maintained at a 70 percent level.

At the other end of the spectrum, another man reported a reduction in excess sleep. The problem had been present for four months. He had also experienced a feeling of heaviness during the day, along with procrastination and lethargy.

Beginning the night of his consultation, he started sleeping two or two and a half hours less each night. He also woke up feeling more refreshed, and felt more focused and clear in activity. The feeling of heaviness has not returned after three months, and he still reports greater vitality, which he attributes to more efficient sleep as a result of his consultation.

This kind of thing is not isolated to this particular ailment. There are many ailments that have been treated successfully by MVVT. You may not have many of these, but there is a good chance that you have some of them, as corollaries to your underlying fatigue.

Musculo-Skeletal Disorders
Osteoarthritis
Rheumatoid Arthritis
Spondylitis
Frozen Shoulder
Back Pain
Disk-Related Problems
Stress Fracture
Sciatica
Heel Spurs

Pain as the Primary Problem
Tension Headache
Migraine Headache
Other Headache
Pain Syndrome
Neuralgia
Carpal Tunnel Syndrome
Pain Following Herpes Zoster
Pain from Cancer

Gastrointestinal Disorders
Digestive Problems
Anorexia
Gastritis
Colitis
Irritable Bowel Syndrome
Constipation
Dysentery
Hyperacidity
Gastric Ulcer
Duodenal Ulcer
Heartburn
Liver Enlargement
Hepatitis A
Anemia

Ano-Rectal Problems
Hemorrhoids
Anal Fissure

Respiratory Disorders
Asthma
Bronchitis
Sinusitis

Skin Disorders
Psoriasis
Eczema
Atopic Dermatitis
Burning and/or Itching Sensations

Cardiovascular Diseases
Stable Angina
Ectopic Heart Beat (heart palpitations)
Hypertension
Peripheral Vascular Disease

Mental Disorders
Insomnia
Anxiety
Depression
Forgetfulness
Anger
Emotional Instability
Grief
Phobia

Eye Problems
Itching or redness
Pain
Pressure
Fatigue
Eye Problems Due to Systemic Illness
Visual Weakness

Gynecological Disorders
Menstrual Disorders
Premenstrual Syndrome
Gynecological Problems
Menopausal Difficulties
Uterine Fibroids (benign uterine tumors)

Numbness
Paralysis

Endocrine Disorders
Diabetes
Thyroid Problems
Adrenal Gland Problems
Kidney Disorder

Immunological Disorders
Allergy

Other Problems
General Weakness
Chronic Fatigue Syndrome
Vertigo (dizziness)
Inflammation of the Glands
Ringing of the Ears (tinnitus)
Prostatitis
Tonsilitis
Kidney Stones
Parkinson's Disease
Benign Tumors
Dental Related
Wounds

Ear and Hearing Problems
Ear Infection
Hearing Problems
Cancer

You might ask what will happen when you get this treatment. During your initial consultation, you will be meeting with a Maharishi Vedic Vibration Technology expert. The expert will then administer specific Vedic vibrations that are traditionally said to restore order to the physiology, by enlivening the inner intelligence of the body on the most fundamental level of sound.

Depending upon the health condition being addressed, you might be asked to lie down, sit or stand. For most ailments, you will not be required to do anything except relax. Many people have commented on how enjoyable, relaxing and pleasant the experience is.

At this point, the expert whispers within himself or herself some specific sounds traditionally chosen for the indicated health concerns and then administers them by blowing on and/or touching the affected area of your body. In some cases, you may be asked to remove an article of clothing or partially disrobe to expose the affected area to the vibration.

Through this procedure, the influence of the sound or vibration permeates the body and enlivens its inner intelligence and self-repair mechanism, bringing about balance to the indicated areas of need. The emphasis of this program is on enlivening the body's inner intelligence to enable the body to heal itself.

That's it. Many people have fascinating results from this simple, yet profound procedure.

Here's a few other points about the treatment from the Vedic Vibration website (www.VedicVibration.com), in a question and answer format.

Will I need to discuss my health concerns during the consultation?

No. All the information about your health concerns needed for your consultation is provided before the consultation in your application form. Your application will be reviewed by an international panel of experts in Maharishi Vedic Vibration Technology who will develop your individualized consultation program. The Vedic Vibration expert that you will meet with will administer the consultation according to this individualized program. The consultation session itself will proceed primarily in quietness.

Many participants have expressed appreciation for the simplicity and profundity of the Maharishi Vedic Vibration Technology sessions. They were pleased that discussion of their health concerns was not required, nor were invasive or uncomfortable diagnostic procedures or treatments involved.

How long does a consultation take? How many days will I need to be available?

One consultation consists of three separate sessions with the Maharishi Vedic Vibration Technology expert. Generally, each session takes 30 to 90 minutes, depending upon the number of disorders being addressed. Consultation sessions may be scheduled on consecutive days or several days apart.

Do I learn anything that I need to practice at home?

This program does not involve learning a technique, listening to audiotapes, or any other practice. In some cases, Maharishi Vedic Vibration Technology works instantaneously to enliven the inner intelligence of the physiology in areas where disorder may be present. That is why this technology is sometimes also referred to as the Instant Relief program.

Who are the Maharishi Vedic Vibration experts?

The Maharishi Vedic Vibration Technology experts are specially trained under the guidance of Maharishi Mahesh Yogi in the application of specific Vedic sounds for specific disorders.

Will I also be meeting with a medical doctor?

It is not necessary for you to meet with a medical doctor as part of the Maharishi Vedic Vibration Technology session. A medical doctor may, however, be evaluating the program in your location for the purpose of determining the effectiveness of this non-medical approach to improving the health of individuals with chronic disorders.

Is the relief that a person gains permanent? Or would someone typically come back every so often for additional sessions?

Most commonly, we observe that the degree of relief a person gains from the consultation remains fairly stable over time if they maintain a healthy routine. However, depending upon the duration and severity of the condition, more than one consultation may be necessary to bring the desired degree of relief. Conditions continue to improve even after the consultation is over.

Is there anything I can do to gain the greatest benefit from my consultation?

This is a very practical and important question. First of all, be prepared to get extra rest: both immediately after your Maharishi Vedic Vibration Technology session, and by going to bed early in the weeks following your consultation.

Another practical suggestion is that, for several days or weeks after your consultation, you avoid activities that could put undue strain on the area of the physiology addressed in your consultation. Along with plenty of rest, a wholesome and balanced diet and a good daily routine, this extra care will give your body the time to gradually stabilize the improvement, and bring maximum benefit from your consultation.

That's the overview, and as we said, it's all about memory. You may not remember every thing that you've read here, but that is not the point. The information that you need is not in this book. It's in your physiology, your DNA, it's the fundamental true sound of your physiology, unencumbered by imbalances, add-ons, stress and strain. It's the memory of who you really are.

You've read this far. You've taken the first step. Why not keep walking, following the memory of that inner melody, all the way home?

Final Note:

Now that the seed of this vast knowledge has been planted in you, it is important to make sure that it grows into a mighty tree and gives you the fruit of health and healing. You might be overwhelmed by the amount of knowledge but once you have grasped the knowledge, then going for the treatment and experience becomes easier. No Vedic expert will be able to give you this much knowledge when you have a consultation, on any level. There is a lot of self help material here and this book will become a guide to take the subsequent steps in expanding your health and consciousness.

You have now understood that you are the wholeness, the wholeness and the totality of all of Nature and consciousness. Any influences on the level of the body, mind, emotions, intellect, behavior, environment and consciousness are all involved in creating imbalance or balance. So slowly but surely you will see healing, health and evolution in all these areas. That is why Maharishi Ayurveda is called consciousness-based medicine and enlightened health. This enlightenment is inevitable because the intellect becomes clear and pure and it will be able to make the right choices which will be not just on an individual level but on a cosmic level.

However, first things first, it is absolutely important that you start feeling good in body and mind so please consult a Maharishi Ayurveda physician and follow the guidelines and the prescription he or she gives you. Many years of studying, practicing and the vast experience gained by the physician are extremely valuable in making the program simple and easy for you. You have to be able to handle it, follow it and get better soon.

I felt so confident with my patients with Maharishi Ayurveda that I even began a campaign that one visit is all you need. For many clients, literally I would only see them once or twice, depending on the severity of the problems. Then if any problems continued and they needed more guidance, I was able to speak to them or email them and guide them into the next course of action. This is how powerful this timeless science can be.

Some of you might be taking conventional medicine and may be under different treatment protocols. You needn't worry that Maharishi Ayurveda protocols and preparations will create side effects or interactions. MA is compatible with conventional medicine and under expert care there are no side effects or the creation of new disease. The physician will be able to guide you how both of them can be utilized for the best outcome and gradually wean you off the conventional medicine if there is no need for it. Or put you on a very small dose just to ensure stability in the treatment process.

Once you feel better, then the whole world looks different. For some of you, chronic fatigue can be completely history and for some of you, the road to recovery is definite, although slower and with some obstacles in the path. Everything really depends on the complexity of the imbalances. This gives an enormous hope and your life will be more fulfilling and enjoyable, with a new level of energy and health. And who knows, at some point we can all join hands to give more positive energy to this world by helping and inspiring others. Each of our contributions is imperative at this moment for our dear world family.

GLOSSARY

abhayanga Ayurvedic oil Massage

agni digestive fire; also the element of fire generally (see *bhutagni, dhatuagni and jatharagni*)

akasha the element of space(see *mahabhuta*)
ama the sticky , bad smelling , toxic remains of undigested food that obstructs the channels in the body

apagni one of the five *bhutagnis*, it helps break down of watery food

Apana Vata one of the five *subdoshas* of **Vata**, governing all downward motion in the body, particularly in lower abdomen
asanas neuromuscular integration exercises

asthi dhatu of the seven *dhatu*'s, asthi is the bone tissue

asthi agni one of the seven *dhatu agnis* . The dhatu agnis transform one tissue into the other in the process of digestion
Avalambaka Kapha one of the five *subdoshas* of the *Kapha*, centered in the chest , heart and lower body; supports physical strength, the back and stamina; regulates moisture in the lungs

Ayurveda "Knowledge of Life span"; a major category of Vedic literature dealing with medicine and health

Bhrajaka Pitta one of the five *subdoshas* of *Pitta*, associated with the skin, including appearance and absorptive activity

bhutagni general term for five types of digestive fire (*agnis*) that correspond with each of the five elements of Nature (earth, water, fire, air, space) and help to digest foods according to the presence of those elements

Bodhaka Kapha one of the five *subdhoshas* of *Kapha*, located in the tongue and throat; regulates secretions in the mouth as well as the sense of taste

Charaka Samhita one of the 40 aspects of Vedic literature; the best known of the six aspects that deal explicitly with medicine and health

deha prakriti one's doshic constitution at any particular point in life (see *dosha, prakriti*)

dhatu any of the seven tissues that make up the body

dhatu agni digestive or metabolic fire associated with each of the seven bodily tissues

dosha any of the three fundamental operators underlying all aspects of mind-body (see *Vata, Pitta*, and *Kapha*)

dravyaguna "qualities of matter"; sophisticated science of preparing Ayurvedic herbal compounds

Gandharva Veda music of the ancient Vedic civilization; the eternal rhythms and melodies of Nature
ghee clarified butter

jala the element of water (see *mahabhuta*)

Janma prakriti the type of mind-body constitution one is born with *jatharagni* the primary digestive fire functioning in the digestive juices in the large and the small intestines and stomach, which are responsible for converting food into the nutrient plasma   that nourishes all the cells and tissues throughout the body; made up of five *bhutagnis*

Jyotish aspect of Vedic Literature concerned with Vedic astrology

Kapha one of the three mind-body operators (*doshas*); governs physical structure, including bones, muscle, and lymphatic system, and fluid balance; primarily situated in the chest; primary qualities: heavy, oily, slow, cold, steady, solid, dull, soft, sweet and smooth

Kayachikitsa "therapy of fire" the field of internal medicine used in Maharishi Rejuvenation therapy to sustain and balance the digestive fire (*agni*), including panchkarma and other procedures (such as *abhayanga*) to purify and pacify the *doshas*

Kledaka Kapha one of the five *subdoshas* of *Kapha*, located in the stomach; responsible for initial phases of digestion, especially moistening the food

mahabhuta any of the basic building blocks or elements of the materials world :earth (*prithivi*), water(*jala*), fire(*tejas*), air (*vayu*), and space(*akasha*)

Maharishi Ayurveda health care program Ayurvedic science of health and system of medicine revived in its completeness by Maharishi Mahesh Yogi

Maharishi Jyotish Program science of prediction   Vedic astrology revived in its completeness by Maharishi Mahesh Yogi

Maharishi Sthapatya Veda Design aspect of Maharishi Vedic Science that includes the health effects of the orientation , design , proportion, and positioning of buildings ; the most ancient and supreme system of country , town, village , and home planning in harmony with Natural Law

majja dhatu one of the seven *dhatus*, majja includes bone marrow and tissues of nervous system

majja agni one of the seven *dhatu agnis*. The dhatu agnis transform one tissue into the other in the process of digestion

mala any of the several types of normal waste produced during formation of the *dhatus*, including urine, feces, sweat, phlegm, bile and various other excreta

mamsa dhatu of the seven *dhatus*, mamsa is muscle tissue

mamsa agni one of the seven *dhatu agnis*. The dhatu agnis transform one tissue into the other in the process of digestion

meda dhatu of the seven *dhatus*, meda is fat tissue

meda agni one of the seven *dhatu agnis*. The dhatu agnis transform one tissue into the other in the process of digestion

ojas the most refined and nourishing product of digestion; the finest material form of consciousness

Osteoporosis a medical condition characterized by a loss of bone density; "brittle bone" disease

Pachaka Pitta one of the five *subdoshas* of *Pitta,* governing digestive secretions in the area of small intestine, duodenum, and lower stomach

pandit an expert thoroughly trained to use Vedic technologies of sound and action to restore the functioning of Natural Law through, for example, the precise performances of *yagyas*

Pitta one of three *doshas;* governs heat, metabolism, and energy production; primarily situated in the area around the navel; primary qualities: hot, sharp, light, acidic, slightly oily, liquid and flowing

pragya-aparadh "mistake of the intellect"

Prana Vata one of the five *subdoshas* of *Vata,* governing movement of air etc., in the head and chest, as well as mental clarity and sensory perception

pranayama neurorespiratory technique involving simple, rhythmic breathing exercises to balance, relax and revitalize the mind-body

prithivi the element of earth (see *mahabhuta*)

prithivi agni one of the five *bhutagnis,* it helps break down of heavy, solid foods

raga musical patterns (melodies) structured according to the principles of *Gandharva Veda* music

rakta dhatu of the seven *dhatus*, rakta equates with blood
Rakta agni one of the seven *dhatu agnis*. The dhatu agnis transform one tissue into the other in the process of digestion

Ranjaka Pitta one of the *subdoshas* of *Pitta,* governing blood chemistry and color from the liver and spleen
rasa essence or taste

rasa dhatu of the seven *dhatus*, rasa is associated with chyle, or plasma, and is the first product of digestion

rasa agni one of the seven *dhatu agnis*. The dhatu agnis transform one tissue into the other in the process of digestion

rishi wise person, enlightened teacher

Sadhaka Pitta one of the *subdoshas* of *Pitta*, located in the heart and associated with desiring, fulfilling desires, memory, enthusiasm and energy

sama-doshas a rare mind-body type characterized by a balance of all three *doshas Vata, Pitta* and *Kapha*

Sama Veda one of the four *Vedas* (Rk, Sama, Yajur and Atharva), whose frequencies express the "flowing wakefulness" quality of Natural Law

Samana Vata one of the five *subdoshas* of *Vata*, located in umbilical region; associated with appetite, production of digestive enzymes, and movement of food through the stomach and intestines

Shleshaka Kapha one of the five *subdoshas* of *Kapha*, responsible for lubrication of joints

shukra the subtlest of the seven *dhatus*; reproductive tissues

srota channels and microchannels within the body, such as veins, arteries and capillaries
Sthapatya Veda aspect of Vedic literature concerned with architecture

Surya namaskara "Salute to the sun" a special sequence of *asanas*, or neuromuscular integration exercises

Tarpaka Kapha one of the five *subdoshas* of *Kapha*, located in the head and cerebrospinal fluid; responsible for nourishing and lubricating the organs of the head and for nourishing the sensory and cognitive faculties and motor organs

tejas the element of fire, also called agni (see *mahabhuta*)

tejas-agni one of the five *bhutagnis*, it helps break down spicy and hot foods

Udana Vata one of the five *subdoshas* of *Vata*, located in throat, chest and navel

vastu correct relationship between a building site and the environment

Vata the "king" of the three mind-body operators(*doshas*), because it leads *Pitta* and *Kapha* in responding to internal and external factors; governs motion of all kinds mental ,physical, emotional from its primary seat in colon ; primary qualities: light, dry, cold, airy and moving.

Vata Kala term used in Vedic texts to refer to the later years of woman's or man's life, characterized by wisdom and tranquility

vayu the element of air (see *mahabhuta*)

Veda "Knowledge"- total knowledge and structure of Natural Law expressed in unmanifest frequencies of sound that precede and produce the physical manifestation of the universe

vikriti a state of imbalance in the doshas characterized by an excess of one or more *doshas*

Vyana Vata one of the five *subdoshas* of *Vata*; governs circulation of blood, lymph, and sweat, as well as nerve impulses promoting , for example, extension and contraction of muscles

yagyas Vedic performances which aim to transform the influences on ones life so as to correct imbalances before they arise

Appendix

Sources for Information on Maharishi Vedic Approach to Health and Related Programs

How to locate a vaidya (ayurvedic expert) in your area
National Tour Center   1-641-209-1981

To contact Kumuda Reddy, M.D.
5009 Paducah road,College Park, MD 20740
www.allhealthyfamily.com
Ph.: 1-866-REDDYMD
1-301-474-2184

CENTERS OFFERING TREATMENT PROGRAMS IN MAHARISHI AYURVEDA

The Raj Maharishi Ayurveda Health Center and Spa   800-248-9050 or
Fairfield, Iowa   641-472-9580
Web site: www.theraj.com

The Maharishi Vedic Health Center   877-890-8600 or
Lancaster, Massachusetts   978-365-4549
Website: http://www.lancasterhealth.com/learn/

Maharishi Vedic Vibration Technology   800-431-9680
Web site: www.vedicvibration.com
E-mail: applications@vedicvibration.com

WHERE TO ORDER MAHARISHI AYUR-VEDA PRODUCTS AND HERBAL FORMULAS

In the United States
Maharishi Ayurveda Products
International, Inc. (MAPI)
402 N. B Street, Fairfield, IA 52556
Web site: www.mapi.com

800-255-8332 or
719-260-55

Get 10% discount on mapi
products by using the code
HP-206-0309 on selected
products - US and Canada
orders only

In Canada
Maharishi Ayurveda Products Canada
Web site: www.mapicanada.ca/index.asp

QUICK REFERENCE GUIDE OF MAHARISHI AYURVEDA PRODUCTS THAT WOULD BE HELPFUL

For Chronic Fatigue

1. Fatigue free
2. Re Gen Vitality
3. Stress free body
4. Stress free mind

For Muscle & Joint Problems

1. Osteo Relief
2. Spice Mix
3. Calcium Support
4. Joint Soothe tablets
5. Joint Soothe II oil

To Balance Digestion

1. Aci - balance
2. Digest Tone
3. Herbal Di- Gest

To Help with Sleep

1. Deep Rest
2. Blissful Sleep
3. Slumber Time Tea
4. Slumber Time Aroma Oil

To Rejunvate the Liver

1. Liver Balance

For Energy & Vitality

1. Stress Free Body
2. ReGen Vitality
3. Vata Tea
4. Stress Free mind

For General Rejuvenation

1. Rejuvenation for Men
2. Rejuvenation for Ladies
3. Vital Lady
4. ReGen Vitality

To Improve Immunity

1. Bio - Immune
2. Amrit

To Detox

1. Elim Tox
2. Elim Tox O
3. Herbal Cleanse
4. Genitrac
5. Mind Flex
6. Worry Free

To Help Balance the Mind & Emotions

1. Mind Plus
2. Stress Free Mind
3. Stress Free Emotions

Please ask Dr Reddy or call MAPI help line as to how to use these and other preparations. To get a 10% discount please use this code HP 206-0309.

TO LOCATE A TEACHER OF THE TRANSCENDENTAL MEDITATION TECHNIQUE IN YOUR AREA

Call toll-free 888-LEARN-TM (888-532-7686)

or see web site: www.tm.org.

FOR INFORMATION AND RESEARCH ON THE TRANSCENDENTAL MEDITATION TECHNIQUE

Information and research on the Transcendental Meditation Technique
www.tm.org

Doctors on the Transcendental Meditation technique and health benefits:
www.doctorsontm.org

The Transcendental Meditation technique and educational benefits:
www.tmeducation.org/
http://adhd-tm.org/

Information for implementing and funding programs for teaching Transcendental Meditation in schools
www.davidlynchfoundation.org
www.cbeprograms.org/ (US)
www.consciousnessbasededucation.org.uk/ (UK)

MAHARISHI SCHOOLS AND UNIVERSITIES

Maharishi School of the Age of Enlightenment
(For Children K-12)
In the United States:
804 North Third Street, Fairfield, IA 52556, 866-472-6723
Fax: 641-472-1211
www.maharishischooliowa.org

Maharishi School of the Age of Enlightenment
(For Children K-12)
In the United Kingdom:
Cobbs Brow Lane, Lathom, Ormskirk, Lancashire, L40 6JJ **UK**
Phone: +44 (0)1695 729912
Fax: +44 (0)1695 729030
www.maharishischool.com

Maharishi University of Management
1000 N. 4th St., Fairfield, IA 52557, (800) 369-6480 or (641) 472-1110
www.mum.edu/

HEALTH EDUCATION COURSES
IN MAHARISHI AYUR-VEDA

Health Education Short Courses:
Full descriptions of these courses can be found at the following web site: www.Maharishi.org.

1. Human Physiology: Expression of Veda and the Vedic Literature
2. Good Health through Prevention
3. The Maharishi Yoga[SM] Program
4. Self-Pulse Reading Course for Prevention
5. Diet, Digestion and Nutrition
6. Maharishi Vedic Astrology Overview
7. Maharishi Vedic Architecture

For training courses in Maharishi Ayur-Veda for physicians and other health professionals:
Maharishi Ayur-Veda Association of America
email: maaa@globalcountry.net
phone (877) 540-6222.

For Degree Programs in Maharishi Integrative Medicine:
Maharishi University of Management
Bachelor's degree and pre-med program, (800) 369-6480 or
(641) 472-1110
E-mail: admissions@mum.edu
Web site: www.mum.edu/premed/

THE MAHARISHI VEDIC ASTROLOGY AND MAHARISHI YAGYA PROGRAMS IN THE UNITED STATES AND CANADA

Maharishi Vedic Astrology and Maharishi Yagya programs
websites: www.maharishiyagya.org
                www.globalgoodfortune.com

For more information, choose the Time Zone you live in:
Time Zone 9 Eastern States (CT, DC, DE, FL, GA, MA, ME, MD, NJ, NC, NH, NY, OH, PA, RI, SC, VA, VT, WV)
530-877-8332 (phone) 530-327-7736 (fax)
maharishiyagyatz9@maharishi.net

Time Zone 10 Central States (AL, AZ, AR, CO, ID, IL, IN, IA, KS, KY, LA, MI, MN, MS, MO, MT, NE, NM, ND, OK, SD, TN, TX, UT, WI, WY)
503-639-0464 (phone) 503-639-3860 (fax)
maharishiyagyatz10@maharishi.net

Time Zone 11 Western States (AK, CA, HI, NV, OR, WA)
530-877-8332 (phone) 530-327-7736 (fax)
maharishiyagyatz11@maharishi.net

(**Outside the U.S.A. and Canada,** please contact the Maharishi Yagya program's international office in Switzerland at +4141-825-1525 phone, +4141-825-1526 fax, jyotish-yagya@maharishi.net email.)

MAHARISHI VEDIC ARCHITECTURE, MAHARISHI VASTU AND THE MAHARISHI STHAPATYA VEDA PROGRAM

Fortune Creating Homes and Communities
www.fortunecreatingbuildings.com
641-472-7570

Recommended Books

Books by Maharishi Mahesh Yogi

Life Supported by Natural Law. Washington, D.C.: Age of Enlightenment Press, 1986.

Age of Enlightenment Publications, 1995.

Maharishi Mahesh Yogi on the Bhagavad-Gita: A New Translation and Commentary, Chapters 1-6. New York: Penguin Books, 1973.

Maharishi Vedic University: Introduction. India: Age of Enlightenment Publications, 1995.

Science of Being and Art of Living. New York: Penguin Books, 1995.

Scientific Research on Maharishi Vedic Approach to Health

Scientific Research on Maharishi's Transcendental Meditation and TM-Sidhi Program: Collected Papers, Volumes 16, available through Maharishi University of Management Press, Press Distribution, DB 1155, Fairfield, Iowa 52557.

Scientific Research on the Maharishi Transcendental Meditation and TM-Sidhi Programs: A Brief Summary of 500 Studies. Fairfield, Iowa: Maharishi University of Management Press, 1996.

Other Books

Deans, Ashely, Ph.D. A Record of Excellence: The Remarkable Success of Maharishi School of the Age of Enlightenment. Septermber, 2005.

Denniston, Denise. The TM Book: How to Enjoy the Rest of Your Life. Fairfield, Iowa: Fairfield Press, 1986.

Nader, Tony, M.D., Ph.D. Human Physiology: Expression of Veda and the Vedic Literature. Vlodrop, The Netherlands: Maharishi Vedic University Press, 2001.

Pearson, Craig, Ph.D. The Complete Book of Yogic Flying. Fairfield, Iowa: Maharishi University of Management Press, 2008.

Reddy, Kumuda, M.D., Egenes, Linda, and Mullins, Margaret, MSN,FNP. For a Blissful Baby: Happy and Healthy Pregnancy through Maharishi Vedic Medicine. Schenectady: New York. Samhita Productions, 1999.

Reddy, Kumuda, M.D.,Stan Kendz. Forever Healthy – Introduction to Maharishi Ayur-Veda Health Care

Reddy, Kumuda, M.D., Linda Egenes. Conquering Chronic Disease –

Through Maharishi Vedic Medicine.

Reddy, Kumuda, M.D., Janardhan Reddy MD with Sandra Willbanks. Golden Transition — Menopause Made Easy through Maharishi Vedic Medicine

Reddy, Kumuda, M.D., Cynthia Lane. Living life free from pain - Treating Arthritis, Joint Pain, Muscle Pain and Fibromyalgia with Maharishi Ayurveda

Reddy, Kumuda, M.D., and Linda Egenes. Super Healthy Kids - A Parents Guide to Maharishi Ayurveda.

Reddy, Kumuda, M.D., Ayurvedic Cooking Made Easy - 100+ Recipes for a Healthy You

Roth, Robert. Maharishi Mahesh Yogi's Transcendental Meditation. New York: Donald I. Fine, 1994.

Schneider, Robert, M.D., Total Heart Health: How to Prevent and Reverse Heart Diseasee with the Maharishi Vedic Approach to Health. Laguna Beach:CA. Basic Health Publications, 2006.

Wallace, R. Keith. The Neurophysiology of Enlightenment. Fairfield, Iowa: Maharishi International University Press, 1986.

Wallace, R. Keith. The Physiology of Consciousness. Fairfield, Iowa: Maharishi International University Press, 1993.

These books and others are available from
Maharishi University of Management Press   800-831-6523
Press Distribution DB 1155
Fairfield, Iowa 52557
E-mail: mumpress@mum.edu
Web site: www.mumpress.com/

A selection of books is also available from Maharishi Ayurveda
Products International (see information above).

www.ingramcontent.com/pod-product-compliance
Lightning Source LLC
Chambersburg PA
CBHW071407170526
45165CB00001B/201